S I R T F O O D D I E T

THE ULTIMATE STEP BY STEP GUIDE FOR FAST WEIGHT LOSS, BURN FAT AND HEAL YOUR BODY. INCLUDES HEALTHY AND TASTY RECIPES FOR YOUR MEAL PLAN

Gregory Matthew

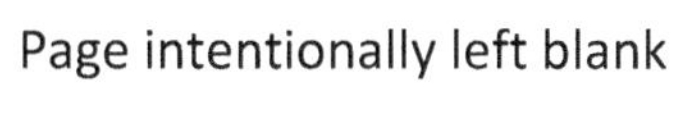

Page intentionally left blank

CONTENT

THE SCIENCE OF SIRTFOOD DIET **6**

 The Change to Sirtfoods 7

 About the Diet 9

 Who Is the Sirtfood Diet Good For? 12

CHAPTER TWO **13**

AN EXPLANATION ABOUT SIRT DIET AND WHY IT WORKS **13**

 The Diet 14

 Step by Step Instructions to Follow the Sirtfood Diet 16

 Is It Healthy and Sustainable? 19

 Safety and Side Effects 21

 Sirtuins Activate Your Body's Wellness Genes 25

 What Foods Enact Sirtuins? 29

 How the Sirtfoods Diet Functions 30

 A Sirtfood Diet Meal Plan 31

 What Would You Be Able to Eat on the Sirtfood Diet? 33

CHAPTER THREE **37**

HEALTH BENEFITS OF SIRTFOOD DIET **37**

Sirtfood Meal Plans ... 38

Foods You Can Eat ... 39

Is Diet Working? ... 40

What the Sirtfood Diet Does. ... 49

What is Matcha? ... 49

Superfood Benefits of Matcha ... 51

CHAPTER FOUR ... 57

A SIMPLE WEEKLY GUIDE THAT FOLLOWS YOU DAY AFTER DAY ... 57

Week 1 ... 58

Weeks 2 and 3 ... 59

Sirtfood green juice (Serves 1) ... 60

Prawn Stir-fry with Noodles (Serves 1) ... 61

Hamburger with red wine, onion rings, and herb simmered potatoes (serves 1) ... 63

Tuscan bean stew (Serves 1) ... 65

The best method to Meal Prep You Week of Meals: ... 66

The sirtfood list ... 75

CHAPTER FIVE ... 77

TOP SIRTFOODS- 20 FOODS THAT ACTIVATE WEIGHT LOSS ... 77

Sirtfood Diet Green Juice ... 81

Sirtfoods with Other Foods ... 83

Sirtfood - What are Medjool Dates? ... 88

Step by Step Instructions to Enjoy Medjool Dates ... 90

CHAPTER SIX ... 94

HOW TO FOLLOW THE SIRTFOOD DIET ... 94

How Can It Work? ... 98

CHAPTER SEVEN ... 101

PHASES OF SIRTFOOD DIET ... 101

Phase 1 of the Sirtfood Diet ... 103

Phase 2 of the Sirtfood Diet ... 103

Phase 1: 7 Pounds in Seven Days ... 105

Step by Step Instructions to Follow Phase 1   107

Phase 2: Maintenance   115

Step by Step Instructions to Follow Phase 2   117

Coming back To Three Meals   120

Sirtfood Bites   122

"Sirtifying" Your Meals   124

Cooking for More   126

A 7-Day Sirtfood Diet Plan – Phase 1 and Phase 2   128

Are Sirtfoods The New Superfoods?   130

Who Shouldn't Try the Sirtfood Diet?   132

Sirtfood Recipes   133

Significant Questions Addressed Often   135

CHAPTER EIGHT   **138**

AFTER THE DIET   **138**

Step by Step Instructions to Maintain Weight Loss After a Diet   138

Ten Habits to Help You Maintain Your Weight   139

CHAPTER NINE   **143**

RECIPES   **143**

Sirtfood Juice   143

Sirt Muesli   145

Fragrant Chicken Bosom With Kale, Red Onions, Tomato and Stew Salsa   146

Sirtfood Nibbles   148

Asian Ruler Prawn Pan Sear With Buckwheat Noodles   150

Strawberry Buckwheat Tabouleh   151

Marinated Baked Cod With Stir-Fried Greens   153

Sirtfood Bites   155

Sirt Super Salad   156

Sweet-smelling Chicken Breast with Kale and Red Onions and a Tomato and Chili Salsa   157

Asian Shrimp Stir-Fry With Buckwheat Noodles   160

Strawberry Buckwheat Tabbouleh   162

Sirtfood Green Juice   163

MIXED OMELET TOAST TOPPER   165

ONE-DISH SUMMER EGGS   166

VEGGIE LOVER COOK   167

COCONUT AND BANANA SANDWICHES   169

SUMMER PORRIDGE   171

VEGETARIAN TOMATO AND CORIANDER HOTCAKES   172

VEGETARIAN GRANOLA   174

MEXICAN BEANS AND AVOCADO TOAST   175

THREE-GRAIN PORRIDGE   176

DAYLIGHT SMOOTHIE   177

VEGGIE LOVER SMOOTHIE   178

KIWI ORGANIC PRODUCT SMOOTHIE   179

THE SIRTFOOD DIET SALMON SUPER-SERVING OF MIXED GREENS   179

THE SIRTFOOD DIET GREEN JUICE SALAD   181

CHICKEN CURRY   182

PREPARED POTATOES WITH SPICY CHICKPEA STEW   184

KALE AND RED ONION DHAL WITH BUCKWHEAT   187

RULER PRAWN STIR FRY WITH BUCKWHEAT NOODLES   189

TURMERIC CHICKEN AND KALE SALAD WITH HONEY LIME DRESSING   191

BUCKWHEAT NOODLES WITH CHICKEN KALE AND MISO DRESSING   194

ASIAN KING PRAWN STIR-FRY WITH BUCKWHEAT NOODLES   196

HEATED SALMON SALAD WITH CREAMY MINT DRESSING   198

CHOC CHIP GRANOLA   200

FRAGRANT ASIAN HOTPOT   202

BUTTERNUT SQUASH AND DATE TAGINE   203

PRAWN ARRABBIATA   207

TURMERIC BAKED SALMON   209

CROWNING CEREMONY CHICKEN SALAD   211

HEATED POTATOES WITH SPICY CHICKPEA STEW-SIRTFOOD RECIPES   212

RED ONION DHAL AND KALE WITH BUCKWHEAT-SIRTFOOD   214

CHARGRILLED BEEF WITH GARLIC KALE, A RED WINE JUS, ONION RINGS, AND HERB ROASTED

POTATOES-SIRTFOOD   217

KALE AND BLACKCURRANT SMOOTHIE   219

BUCKWHEAT PASTA SALAD   220

Greek Salad Skewers — 221

Kale, Edamame and Tofu Curry — 222

Chocolate Cupcakes with Matcha Icing — 224

Sesame Chicken Salad — 226

Sirtfood Mushroom Scramble Eggs — 228

Sweet-smelling Chicken Breast with Kale, Red Onion, and Salsa — 229

Smoked Salmon Omelet — 231

Green Tea Smoothie — 232

Sirtfood Marinated Cod with Sesame — 233

Raspberry and Blackcurrant Jelly — 234

Apple Pancakes with Blackcurrant Compote — 236

Sirt Fruit Salad — 237

Sirtfood Bites — 238

Sirt Muesli — 240

Chinese-Style Pork with Pak Choi — 241

Tuscan Bean Stew — 244

THE SCIENCE OF SIRTFOOD DIET

The advancement came when it was ound that the advantages of fasting were facilitated by actuating our old sirtuin qualities, otherwise called the "slim gene." At the point when vitality is hard to come by, precisely as found in calorie limitation, an expanded measure of pressure is put on our cells. This is detected by the sirtuins, which at that point, get turned on and communicate incredible signs that fundamentally adjust how our cells act.

Sirtuins increase the digestion, increment the productivity of muscles, switch on fat consumption, decrease inflammation, and fix any harm in cells. As a result, sirtuins make us fitter, more slender, and more advantageous.

The Change to Sirtfoods

"Sirtfoods" are the historical methods for enacting our sirtuin qualities in an ideal manner. These are the marvel foods, especially wealthy in explicit common plant synthetic compounds, called polyphenols, which have the ability to address our sirtuin qualities, turning them on. Generally, they emulate the impacts of fasting and practice and, in doing so, bring amazing advantages by helping the body to all the more likely control glucose levels, consume fat, form muscle and lift wellbeing and memory.

Since they're fixed, plants have built up an exceptionally modern pressure reaction system and produce polyphenols to assist them with adjusting to the difficulties of their condition. At the point when we expend these plants, we additionally devour these polyphenol supplements. Their impact is significant: they actuate our natural pressure reaction pathways.

While all plants have reaction systems, just certain ones have created to deliver critical measures of sirtuin-initiating polyphenols. These plants are sirtfoods. Their revelation implies that rather than severe fasting regimens or rigorous exercise programs, there's currently a progressive better approach to initiate your sirtuin qualities: eating a diet copious in sirtfoods. The best part is that this one includes putting (sirt) foods onto your plate, not taking them off.

Created by two UK-based men with graduate degrees in medicine, the diet has gotten famous among big names and competitors in the UK. Both Pippa Middleton and Adele are supposed to have followed this plan. In the same way as other different diets, the Sirtfood Diet touts compelling and continued weight loss, mind-boggling vitality, and gleaming wellbeing. However, is the Sirtfood Diet another diet trend, or is there any reality to its cases?

About the Diet

The plan guarantees that eating certain foods will enact your "thin quality" pathway and make them shed seven pounds in seven days. Foods like kale, dim chocolate, and wine contain a special concoction called polyphenols that mirror the impacts of activity and fasting. Strawberries, red onions, cinnamon, and turmeric are likewise amazing sirtfoods. These foods will activate the sirtuin pathway to assist the trigger with weighting loss. The science sounds tempting, yet in all actuality, there's little research to back up these cases. Also, the guaranteed pace of weight loss in the first week is relatively speedy and not following the National Institute of Health's safe weight loss rules of one to two pounds every week.

The diet has two phases:
Phase 1 keeps going for seven days. For the initial three days, you drink three sirtfood green juices and one meal rich in sirtfoods for an aggregate of about 1,000 calories. On days four through seven, you drink two green juices and two snacks for a total of 1,500 calories.

Phase 2 is a 14-day upkeep plan, even though it is intended for you to shed pounds consistently (not keep up your present weight). Every day comprises of three adjusted sirtfood meals and one green juice.

After these three weeks, you're urged to keep eating a diet rich in sirtfoods and drinking a green squeeze day by day. You can discover a few sirtfood cookbooks on the web and recipes on the sirtfood site. Green juice recipe found on the sirtfood site comprises of a combo of kale and other verdant greens, parsley, celery, green apple, ginger, lemon juice, and matcha. Buckwheat and lovage are additional ingredients that are suggested for use in your green juice. The diet suggests that juices ought to be made in a juicer, not a blender, so it tastes better.

A day on the sirtfood diet may resemble this:

Breakfast: Soy yogurt with blended berries, cleaved pecans, and dim chocolate

Lunch: A sirtfood plate of mixed greens made with kale,

parsley, celery, apple, pecans beat with olive oil blended in with lemon squeeze and ginger.

Dinner: Stir-seared prawns with kale and buckwheat noodles. Additionally, one sirtfood green juice every day.

The Costs

You truly need to plan and approach the prescribed ingredients to follow this diet appropriately. You'll likewise need to put resources into an excellent juicer, which can cost you at least $100. The regularity of ingredients makes it somewhat intense to get strawberries and kale certain seasons. It's likewise hard to follow when voyaging, at get-togethers, and taking care of a family with little youngsters.

The diet itself removes various food gatherings and is restricting. Dairy foods, which give a variety of essential supplements, including a few that most people need, aren't suggested on the plan. Further, the polyphenol-rich food matcha frequently contains lead in the tea leaves, which is possibly hazardous to your wellbeing, particularly when taken regularly. It additionally has a substantial and unpleasant flavor, as 85% dim chocolate, which is likewise suggested.

Who Is the Sirtfood Diet Good For?

Even though the beginning time of the Sirtfood diet of squeezing and fasting appears to be only useful for the individuals who should lose a little weight rapidly, the abrogating point of the Sirtfood diet is to incorporate more advantageous foods into your diet to build your prosperity and lift your safe system. However, there is an increasingly significant objective. While the initial seven days may appear to be troublesome, the more drawn out term plan can work for everybody.

By concentrating on bringing Sirtfood rich ingredients into your everyday meals, you can proceed with the fat consumption while making the most of your ordinary top picks. This is an eating plan that can keep on bringing benefits over a protracted period.

CHAPTER TWO

AN EXPLANATION ABOUT SIRT DIET AND WHY IT WORKS

The Sirtfood diet stays a hotly debated issue and includes supporters receiving a diet rich in 'sirtfoods.' As per the diet's originators, these different foods work by initiating specific proteins in the body called sirtuins. Sirtuins are accepted to shield cells in the body from passing on when they are under pressure and are thought to control inflammation, digestion, and the maturing procedure. It's the idea that sirtuins impact the body's capacity to consume fat and lift metabolism, bringing about a seven-pound weight loss a week while looking after muscle. In any case, a few specialists accept this is probably not going to be an exclusively fat loss; however, it will instead reflect changes in glycogen stores from skeletal muscle and the liver.

The Diet

So what are these otherworldly 'sirtfoods'? The ten most regular include:

- Green tea
- Dark chocolate (that is in any event 85 percent cocoa)
- Apples
- Citrus natural products
- Parsley
- Turmeric
- Kale
- Blueberries
- Capers
- Red wine

The diet is separated into two phases; the underlying phase

keeps going one week and includes confining calories to 1000kcal for three days, devouring three sirtfood green juices, and one meal rich in sirtfoods every day. The juices incorporate kale, celery, rocket, parsley, green tea, and lemon. Meals incorporate turkey escalope with sage, tricks and parsley, chicken and kale curry and prawn pan sear with buckwheat noodles. From days four to seven, vitality admissions are expanded to 1500kcal, including two sirtfood green juices and two sirtfood-rich meals a day.

Even though the diet advances healthy foods, it's prohibitive in both your food decisions and everyday calories, particularly during the underlying stages. It additionally includes drinking juice, with the sums recommended during phase one surpassing the present day by day rules.

The subsequent phase is known as the support phase, which keeps going 14 days where consistent weight loss happens. The creators trust it's a practical and reasonable approach to shed pounds. Notwithstanding, concentrating on weight loss isn't what the diet is about – it's intended to be tied in with eating the best foods nature brings to the table. In the long haul, they suggest eating three adjusted sirtfood sumptuous meals a day alongside one sirtfood green juice.

Step by Step Instructions to Follow the Sirtfood Diet

The Sirtfood Diet has two phases that the last aggregate of three weeks. From that point forward, you can keep "sirtifying" your diet by including many sirtfoods as could be expected under the circumstances in your meals. The particular recipes for these two phases are found in The Sirtfood Diet book, which was composed of the diet's creators. You'll have to buy it to follow the diet. The meals are loaded with sirtfoods; however, incorporate different ingredients other than merely the "best 20 sirtfoods."

The majority of the ingredients and sirtfoods are anything but difficult to track down. In any case, three of the mark ingredients required for these two phases — matcha green tea powder, lovage, and buckwheat — might be costly or hard to track down. A significant piece of the diet is its green juice, which you'll have to make yourself somewhere in the range of one and multiple times day by day. You will require a juicer (a blender won't work) and a kitchen scale, as the ingredients are recorded by weight. The recipe is beneath:

Sirtfood Green Juice

- 75 grams (2.5 oz.) kale

- 30 grams (1 oz.) arugula (rocket)

- 5 grams parsley

- 2 celery sticks

- 1 cm (0.5 in) ginger

- Half a green apple

- Half a lemon

A large portion of a teaspoon coordinate a green tea

Squeeze all ingredients aside from the green tea powder and lemon together, and empty them into a glass. Juice the lemon by hand; at that point, mix both the lemon squeeze and green tea powder into your juice.

Phase One

The principal phase keeps going seven days and includes

calorie limitation and heaps of green juice. It is planned to kick off your weight loss and professed to assist you with shedding 7 pounds (3.2 kg) in seven days. During the initial three days of phase one, calorie admission is limited to 1,000 calories. You drink three green juices every day in addition to one meal. Every day you can look over recipes in the book, which all include sirtfoods as a fundamental piece of the meal.

Meal models incorporate miso-coated tofu, the sirtfood omelet, or a shrimp pan sear with buckwheat noodles. On days 4–7 of phase one, calorie admission is expanded to 1,500. This incorporates two green juices for each day and two more sirtfood-rich meals, which you can look over the book.

Phase Two

Phase two goes on for two weeks. During this "support" phase, you should keep on consistently shed pounds. There is no particular calorie limit for this phase. Instead, you eat three meals brimming with sirtfoods and one green juice for each day. Once more, the meals are browsed recipes gave in the book.

After the Diet

You may repeat these two phases as regularly as wanted for additional weight loss. In any case, you are urged to keep "sirtifying" your diet after finishing these phases by consolidating sirtfoods routinely into your meals. There is an assortment of Sirtfood Diet books that are brimming with recipes rich in sirtfoods. You can likewise incorporate sirtfoods in your diet as a tidbit or in recipes you as of now use. Furthermore, you are urged to keep drinking the green squeeze each day. Along these lines, the Sirtfood Diet turns out to be, to a higher degree, a way of life change than a one-time diet.

Is It Healthy and Sustainable?

Sirtfoods are practically all healthy decisions and may even bring about some medical advantages because of their cancer prevention agent or mitigating properties. However, eating only a bunch of exceptionally healthy foods can't meet the entirety of your body's wholesome needs. The Sirtfood Diet is pointlessly prohibitive and offers no reasonable, exceptional medical advantages over some other sort of diet. Moreover, eating just 1,000 calories is commonly not suggested without the oversight of a doctor. In any event, eating 1,500 calories for each day is unnecessarily prohibitive for some individuals.

The diet likewise requires drinking up to three green juices for each day. Even though juices can be a decent wellspring of nutrients and minerals, they are likewise a wellspring of sugar and contain practically none of the healthy fiber that whole foods from the ground do. Also, tasting on juice all through the whole day is an ill-conceived notion for both your glucose and your teeth. Also, because the diet is so constrained in calories and food decisions, it is more than likely lacking in protein, nutrients, and minerals, particularly during the primary phase.

Because of the low-calorie levels and prohibitive food decisions, this diet might be hard to adhere to for the whole three weeks. Add that to the high introductory costs of buying a juicer, the book, and certain uncommon and costly ingredients, just as the time costs of getting ready explicit meals and juices, and this diet gets unfeasible and impractical for some individuals.

The Sirtfood Diet advances healthy foods yet is prohibitive in calories and food decisions. It likewise includes drinking loads of juice, which is not a fit suggestion.

Safety and Side Effects

Even though the primary phase of the Sirtfood Diet is low in calories and healthfully deficient, there are no genuine safety worries for the standard, healthy grown-up thinking about the diet's brief span. However, for somebody with diabetes, calorie limitation, and drinking, for the most part, squeeze for the initial not many days of the diet may cause risky changes in glucose levels. By and by, even a healthy individual may encounter some symptoms — essentially hunger.

Eating just 1,000–1,500 calories for each day will leave pretty much anybody feeling hungry, mainly if a lot of what you're expending is juice, which is low in fiber, a supplement that helps keep you feeling full. During phase one, you may encounter different symptoms, for example, weariness, wooziness, and peevishness because of the calorie limitation.

For the healthy grown-up, positive wellbeing results are far-fetched if the diet is followed for just three weeks. The Sirtfood Diet is low in calories, and phase one isn't healthfully adjusted. It might leave you hungry, yet it's not dangerous for the average healthy grown-up.

Sirtfoods are, for the most part, plant-based and high in cell reinforcements that help stunt your body into consuming fat at a higher rate. It's called Sirt because it incorporates eating foods that are high in sirtuin activators, characterized as seven proteins found in the body that direct digestion, inflammation, and the life span of cells. Created by two British Nutritionists, Aidan Goggins and Glen Matten, the foods should initiate your body's "thin quality" to consume fat quicker. They composed a book that is the "official" direct: The Official Sirtfood Diet.

Why it works:

Sirtfoods help signal the body that it should fire up your digestion and increment bulk while you consume fat.

Otherwise called superfoods, the best sirtfoods incorporate the rundown. Note that everybody gets excited about the wine and chocolate; however, your body is very eating more fiber, more cancer prevention agents, and supplement solid foods.

What you can eat:

- Kale

- Red wine

- Strawberries

- Onions

- Garlic

- Soy

- Parsley

- Extra virgin olive oil

- Dark chocolate (85% cocoa)

- Matcha green tea

- Buckwheat

- Turmeric

- Walnuts

- Arugula (rocket)

- Bird's eye stew (peppers)

- Lovage (herb)

- Medjool dates

- Red chicory

- Blueberries

- Capers

- Coffee

The most effective method to start

Week 1. On the Sirtfood diet implies you limit your calorie admission to 1,000 calories per day and drink three Sirtfood green squeezes for the day. The ingredients of a Sirtfood green juice are: Kale, arugula, parsley, celery, including the leaves, a large portion of a green apple, the juice of half of a lemon, and matcha green tea (we like. You can have it over ice or include water; however, don't add plant-based milk or different ingredients not on the list.

Week 2. You should build calories to 1,500 every day, and just beverage two of the Sirtfood Juices a day, also, to have two sirtfood meals every day. Proceed on this example until you have lost the good measure of weight that your body needs to feel your best. A healthy weight loss will include. If you lose 2 to 3 pounds per week, that implies you'll have shed 15 pounds in five weeks

Sirtuins Activate Your Body's Wellness Genes

People groups have consistently been interested in the 'Wellspring of Youth' and how we can live more and more advantageous lives. Established researchers have a similar interest with a group of qualities called sirtuins. All of us houses sirtuins—regularly alluded to as our thin qualities—and they are entrancing, holding the ability to decide things like our capacity to consume fat and remain slim, our weakness to sickness. Even to what extent we can live.

So what makes sirtuins so incredible? Sirtuins are extraordinary as a result of their capacity to change our phones to a sort of endurance mode—setting off a fantastic reusing process that gets out of cell waste and consumes fat. The advantages of this are quite astounding: Fat melts away, and we become fitter, more slender, and more beneficial.

So how would we exploit sirtuins?

This brings up the issue: What would we be able to do to initiate sirtuins and receive these handsome rewards? It is notable that both were fasting and exercise enact sirtuins—however, too bad, both interest a steady promise to either food limitation or requesting exercise systems. Curtailing calories leaves us feeling exhausted, hungry, and irritable, and in the more extended term can prompt muscle loss and stale digestion. Concerning work out, the sum should have been viable for weight loss requires a LOT of exertion. Both can be difficult to achieve.

The aftereffects of one of the most renowned healthful examinations at any point completed were distributed. The reason for the investigation, called PREDIMED, was flawlessly straightforward: It examined the distinction between a Mediterranean-style diet enhanced with either extra-virgin olive oil or nuts and an increasingly traditional present-day diet. Results indicated that following five years, coronary illness and diabetes were sliced by a mind-blowing 30 percent, alongside significant decreases in the danger of obesity in the Mediterranean diet gathering. This wasn't unexpected, yet when the examination was researched in greater detail, it was found there was no distinction in calorie, fat, or starch admission between the two gatherings. How would you clarify that?

Not every (healthy) food are created equivalent.

Research currently shows that plants contain conventional mixes called polyphenols that have enormous advantages for our wellbeing. What's more, when specialists are breaking PREDIMED researched polyphenol utilization among the members, the outcomes were faltering. Over only the five-year time frame, the individuals who expended the most significant levels of polyphenols had 37 percent fewer deaths contrasted with the individuals who ate the least.

In any case, not all polyphenols are equivalent. Information out of Harvard University from more than 124,000 people demonstrated that certain lone polyphenols were useful for weight control. Thus, an investigation of very nearly 3,000 twins found that a higher admission of just certain polyphenols was connected with less muscle to fat ratio and more advantageous dissemination of fat in the body. Polyphenols are, without a doubt, an aid for remaining thin and healthy, yet if not all polyphenols are equivalent, at that point, which is the best? Might it be able to be those that exploration has indicated have the capacity to turn on our sirtuin qualities? The same ones initiated by fasting and exercise?

The pharmaceutical business has rushed to misuse these sirtuin-initiating supplements, contributing several million to change over them into panacea drugs. For instance, well-known diabetes medicates metformin originates from a plant and enacts our sirtuin qualities. However, as of recently, they have been, to a great extent, disregarded by the universe of nourishment, to the hindrance of our wellbeing and our waistlines.

What Foods Enact Sirtuins?

With our advantage provoked, we put all the foods with the most elevated levels of sirtuin-actuating polyphenols together into an extraordinary diet. This incorporates extra-virgin olive oil and pecans, the particular considerations in PREDIMED, just as arugula, red onions, strawberries, red wine, dim chocolate, green tea, and espresso among numerous others. At the point when we pilot tried it, the outcomes were staggering. Members shed pounds, while either keeping up or in any event, expanding their bulk. The best part is that individuals announced inclination great—overflowing with vitality, resting better, and with prominent enhancements in their skin.

Thus, the Sirtfood Diet was conceived, a progressive better approach to enact sirtuins by eating delightful foods. A diet that doesn't include calorie forgetting about, removing carbs, or eating low fat. A menu of incorporation where you receive the rewards from eating the foods your affection. The Sirtfood Diet is stirring things up of healthy eating guidance and what it truly intends to look and feel great. And all from eating our preferred foods!

How the Sirtfoods Diet Functions

Phase one of the Sirtfood diet is the hyper-achievement phase, a clinically demonstrated method for losing a normal of 3.2kg in seven days. During the initial three days, calorie admission is confined to a limit of 1000 calories every day. This comprises of three sirtfood-rich green juices, in addition to one full meal rich in sirtfoods every day. For a considerable length of time, four to seven, calorie admission increments to a limit of 1500 calories. Every day involves two sirtfood-rich green juices and two sirtfood-rich meals.

Phase two is the 14-day upkeep phase, where despite not concentrating on cutting calories, weight is lost consistently. This phase comprises of three adjusted sirtfood-rich meals every day, alongside a "support" sirtfood green juice. The excellence of the Sirtfood diet is that you don't need to be continually dieting. By coordinating more sirtfoods into your everyday diet, you'll be set to receive positive rewards for a fantastic remainder.

A Sirtfood Diet Meal Plan

Because of these standards, this is what could be on the menu longer than a week during the support phase (green squeezes aside).

Breakfast

- Kale omelet

- Muesli, yogurt and blueberries

- Fruit smoothie made with moved oats and soy milk

Lunch and dinner

- Rocket serving of mixed greens with fish, tomatoes, and cucumber wearing olive oil

- Veggie-pressed hot tofu pan sear with feathered creatures eye bean stew

- Grilled fish with buckwheat serving of mixed greens

- Chicken and soba noodle pan sear

- Tofu burgers with wholegrain bread and serving of mixed greens

- Kale serving of mixed greens with edamame beans and red onion wearing olive oil

- Spicy chicken curry presented with wholegrain earthy colored rice

Snacks

- Coffee

- Celery and hummus

- Fresh organic product, especially strawberries, apples, and oranges

- Walnuts

- Dark chocolate

The sirtfood diet rest on the fact that specific foods initiate sirtuins in your body, which are specific proteins theorized to receive different rewards, from shielding cells in your body from inflammation to turning around maturing. Foods permitted on a diet incorporate green tea, dim chocolate, apples, natural citrus products, parsley, turmeric, kale, blueberries, tricks, and red wine.

On the authority sirtfood diet site, advocates clarify that the diet has two "simple" phases. Phase one is seven days with every day comprising of three sirtfood green juices and one meal loaded up with sirtfoods — a sum of 1,000 calories. In any case, don't be disheartened: You may be marginally less starving on days four through seven when you're permitted to build your admission to 1,500 calories with two green juices and two meals. Phew!

Phase two isn't substantially more encouraging. This phase goes on for two weeks, in which you are allowed to have three "adjusted" sirtfood-rich meals every day, notwithstanding your one exceptional green juice. The objective during this time is to advance further weight loss. While the advantages of sirtuins appear to be encouraging, the sirtfood diet is showcased up 'til now another approach to "shed seven pounds in seven days!" And you know at this point extreme diets simply don't work that way.

What Would You Be Able to Eat on the Sirtfood Diet?

The Sirtfood Diet feature grabbers are red wine, and dim

chocolate since the two of them happen to be high in sirtuin activators. Even though that is not the entire picture and you won't feel the impacts by mainlining Merlot and Green and Blacks (more's the pity).

The Sirtfood Diet plan centers on increasing your admission of healthy sirtfoods. These incorporate the accompanying:

- Apples
- Citrus natural products
- Red wine
- Buckwheat
- Walnuts
- Dark chocolate
- Medjool dates
- Parsley
- Capers
- Blueberries
- Green tea
- Soy
- Strawberries

- Tumeric

- Olive oil

- Red onion

- Rocket

- Kale.

Extraordinarily, another top sirtfood is espresso, which is welcome news in case you're exhausted from being advised to remove caffeine. Nations where individuals as of now devour many sirtfoods incorporate Japan and Italy, which are both consistently positioned among the world's most advantageous countries.

Is there a Sirtfood Diet plan?

Indeed, there is.

Week 1

- Limit your admission to 1000 calories per day

- Drink three sirtfood green squeezes a day

- Eat one sirtfood sumptuous meal a day.

Week 2

- Up your admission to 1500 calories per day

- Drink two sirtfood green squeezes a day

- Eat two sirtfood-rich meals a day.

In the long haul, there is no set plan. It's everything about altering your way of life to incorporate; however, many sirtfoods as could be expected under the circumstances, which should cause you to feel more advantageous and progressively vivacious. See point 5 (beneath) for additional subtleties.

Who follows the Sirtfood Diet as of now?

The Sirtfood Diet, as of now, has a developing number of big-name fans, including Adele, Jodie Kidd, Lorraine Pascale, and Sir Ben Ainslie.

CHAPTER THREE

HEALTH BENEFITS OF SIRTFOOD DIET

Creators of the Sirtfood diet say that foods rich in polyphenols (cell reinforcements) turn on "thin" qualities in your body that copy exercise and fasting, kick off weight loss, help digestion, increment disposition and improve maturing. Instances of polyphenol-rich foods the Sirtfood diet urges you to eat incorporate green tea, dim chocolate, espresso, red wine, and kale.

Sirtfood Meal Plans

At the point when you follow the Sirtfood diet, you'll start with phase 1—which goes on for seven days. During the initial three days of the menu, you'll drink three Sirtfood squeezes and have one Sirtfood-rich meal for a day by day aggregate of 1,000 calories. On days four, however, through seven, you'll expend 1,500 complete calories, drink two green squeezes and eat two healthy Sirtfood-rich meals. This finishes at phase 1.

Phase 2 keeps going 14 days and permits you to eat three adjusted Sirtfood-rich meals and one green squeeze day by day. After phase 2 is finished, you'll follow an increasingly typical method of eating—yet are urged to fuse sirtuin-initiating foods into ordinary meal plans. You can reappear phases 1 and 2 whenever you have to lose more weight or muscle to fat ratio.

Foods You Can Eat

You'll presumably need to buy a juicer when following the Sirtfood diet. The accompanying foods and beverages are supported:

- Green juices (containing matcha green tea, lovage and buckwheat)

- Green tea

- Coffee

- Cocoa powder

- Dark chocolate

- Turmeric

- Kale

- Onions

- Parsley

- Ginger

- Olive oil

- Red chicory

- Soy yogurt

- Fruits

- Vegetables

- Walnuts

- Eggs

- Bacon

- Turkey

- Seafood

- Whole-grain pitas

- Cheese

- Hummus

- Buckwheat noodles

- Red wine

Avoid dairy foods when following the Sirtfood diet.

Is Diet Working?

Analysts inspected impacts of Sirtfoods (sirtuin-actuating foods) on wellbeing and weight the board. An audit inferred that polyphenols seem to assist lower with bodying weight, blood glucose, and pulse—yet more research is required here.

The creators of the Sirtfood Diet make intense cases, including that the diet can super-charge weight loss, turn on your "thin quality" and forestall infections. The issue is there isn't a lot of verification to back them. Up until now, there's no persuading proof that the Sirtfood Diet has a more valuable impact on weight loss than some other calorie-confined diet.

Also, albeit a considerable lot of these foods have energizing properties, there have not been any drawn-out human examinations to decide if eating a diet rich in sirtfoods has any substantial medical advantages. The Sirtfood Diet book reports the aftereffects of a pilot study directed by the writers and including 39 members from their wellness place. However, the aftereffects of this examination show up not to have been distributed anyplace else.

For one week, the members followed the diet and practiced day by day. Toward the week's end, members lost a normal of 7 pounds (3.2 kg) and kept up or even picked up the bulk. However, these outcomes are not unusual. Limiting your calorie admission to 1,000 calories and practicing simultaneously will about consistently cause weight loss.

In any case, this sort of brisk weight loss is neither certifiable nor enduring, and this investigation didn't follow members after the first week to check whether they recovered any of the weight, which is ordinarily the situation.

At the point when your body is vitality denied, it goes through its crisis vitality stores, or glycogen, notwithstanding consuming fat and muscle. Every atom of glycogen requires 3–4 particles of water to be put away. At the point when your body goes through glycogen, it disposes of this water too. It's known as "water weight."

In the first week of extraordinary calorie limitation, just around 33% of the weight loss originates from fat, while the other 66% originates from water, muscle, and glycogen. When your calorie admission expands, your body recharges its glycogen stores, and the weight returns right. Lamentably, this sort of calorie limitation can likewise make your body bring dits metabolic rate, causing you to need significantly fewer calories every day for vitality than previously.

This diet may assist you with shedding a couple of pounds

before all else. However, it will probably return when the diet is finished. To the extent of forestalling sickness, three weeks is likely not long enough to have any quantifiable long haul sway. Then again, adding sirtfoods to your ordinary diet over the long haul might just be a smart thought. In any case, you should avoid the diet and begin doing that now. This diet may assist you in getting more fit since it is low in calories; however, the weight is probably going to return once the diet closes. The diet is too short to even think about having a drawn-out effect on your wellbeing.

Specific foods initiate sirtuins in your body, which are specific proteins conjectured to receive different rewards, from shielding cells in your body from inflammation to turning around maturing. Foods permitted on a diet incorporate green tea, dim chocolate, apples, organic citrus products, parsley, turmeric, kale, blueberries, tricks, and red wine.

Lots of persons clarify that the diet has two "simple" phases. Phase one is seven days with every day comprising of three sirtfood green juices and one meal loaded up with sirtfoods —

a sum of 1,000 calories. Yet, don't be debilitated: You may be somewhat less starving on days four through seven when you're permitted to expand your admission to 1,500 calories with two green juices and two meals. Phew!

Phase two isn't considerably more encouraging. This phase goes on for two weeks, in which you are allowed to have three "adjusted" sirtfood-rich meals every day, notwithstanding your one uncommon green juice. The objective during this time is to advance further weight loss. While the advantages of sirtuins appear to be encouraging, the sirtfood diet is showcased up 'til now another approach to "shed seven pounds in seven days!" And you know at this point extraordinary diets simply don't work that way.

Here are three motivations to take a pass on the sirtfood diet:

1. The sirtfood diet estimates achievement just as far as weight loss.
I've said it previously, and I'll state it once more: Weight is a determinant of wellbeing, yet it's not alone. To quantify

somebody's wellbeing accomplishment on whether they lose X pounds in X measure of time overlooks the various advantages of food. Food is loaded with vitality, which permits you to do things like showering, practicing, and breathing. It likewise has supplements that can advance a few real capacities and is regularly a happy encounter established in the convention. For in general wellbeing, there's a great deal more to concentrate on than essential appearance, and estimating achievement just as far as weight loss is incomprehensive.

2. Its prohibitive, which can harm your relationship with food.

This diet accentuates an intake of 1,000 to 1,500 calories every day, which is a lot of lower than a great many people need. At the point when we severely limit our food intake, our natural response is to overeat. Your body is brilliant, and it thinks about this absence of food as an assault. In this manner, we will, in general, overcompensate, which is the reason we as a whole can identify with being "hangry" and thus overindulging whenever we're at long last allowed to eat.

Rehearsing careful and natural eating is a more practical course than confining food.

3. The sirtfood diet isn't science-based.

While there is some dubious research about the advantages of sirtuins, there's almost no exploration about the particular sirtfood diet. Plus, we, as of now, have a few rules set up that have been thoroughly explored and tried for quite a long time. In case you're lost on what "healthy food" is, this is a superior spot to begin.

It's beautiful if you need to join a couple of sirtfoods into an eating plan. Foods like green tea, organic product, dull chocolate, and kale all include a spot inside a healthy eating design! In any case, clinging to a program with such severe pass-or-bomb prerequisites is ridiculous and could be destructive to your relationship with food. By fusing an eating plan that is loaded with assortment and eating carefully, you'll have the option to build up a long haul, solid relationship with food.

- Buckwheat

- Capers

- Celery

- Chilli

- Chocolate

- Coffee

- Extra Virgin Olive Oil

- Green Tea – in a perfect world matcha

- Kale

- Lovage

- Medjool Dates

- Parsley

- Red Chicory

- Red Onion

- Red Wine

- Rocket

- Soy

- Strawberries

- Turmeric

Section 1 of the Sirtfood diet plan is the underlying stage, a method for losing a normal of 3kg in the initial seven days. During the initial three days, calorie admission is set to a limit of 1000 calories each day. This comprises of three sirtfood green juices, in addition to one full meal with sirtfoods every day. For days four to seven, calorie admission is lifted to a limit of 1500 calories. Every day includes two sirtfood green juices and two sirtfood meals.

Section 2 is the 14-day duration phase, where despite not focusing on diminishing calories, weight is decreased steadily. This part comprises of three adjusted sirtfood meals for each day, alongside a sirtfood green juice.

The truth of the Sirtfood diet plan is that you don't need to be always in strict diet mode. By coordinating more sirtfoods into your everyday food intake, you will have the option to pick up the good, healthy focal points for daily living.

What the Sirtfood Diet Does.

Weight loss from fat and not muscle

Lead your body to long haul weight loss achievement

Ensure you look and feel much improved

Give you more vitality

Keeps you from adapting to outrageous fasting and yearning

Allow you to stay away from serious exercise systems

Be a driving force for a more drawn out, more advantageous and infection-free presence

What is Matcha?

Matcha (articulated MA-cha), has been a piece of the Japanese culture since the twelfth century. It is one of the most prized refreshments in Japan. Matcha green tea varies from standard green tea because of how the leaves are delivered. All beverages begin from a similar plant known as Camellia sinensis, which is a bush local to China. The bush offers a wide range of leaves for tea, including white, green oolong, dark, and pu-erh tea. Contingent upon the district and how they're prepared, these kinds of drinks vary in their cancer prevention agent content, their caffeine content.

Difference Between Matcha And Regular Green Tea

Matcha is a kind of tea that is far less handled than customary green tea because the leaves are never heated and held under shade to save the regular supplements found in the leaves. Standard green tea experiences significantly more handling during creation and is additionally left to dry in the sun, versus in the shade like matcha is. Matcha green tea is a brilliant, green powder that is additionally blended into the warmed fluid as opposed to bubbling and fermenting methods utilized when making regular green tea. Since you're expending the leaves entirely in a milder powder with matcha, you're additionally taking in a more significant number of supplements than merely discarding the rest in a tea pack or stressing them out in a sifter as you would with ordinary tea.

How Does Matcha Taste?

Like all green tea, matcha has grass notes marginally, yet with a lot more extravagant, practically rich flavor. It's particularly delicious when mixed with some non-dairy milk and stevia, alongside a little vanilla concentrate.

Superfood Benefits of Matcha

1. Matcha green tea far outranks even probably the most remarkable superfoods we are aware of today. It contains more than multiple times the cell reinforcements in goji berries, numerous times the cancer prevention agents in dim chocolate, numerous times a more significant number of cancer prevention agents than blueberries, and numerous times the cell reinforcements found in spinach. Furthermore, that is simply in one teaspoon!

2. Matcha contains multiple times a more significant amount of the well-known cancer prevention agent EGCG found in customary green tea. EGCG is a piece of the cancer

prevention agent family known as catechins, which have been connected to better heart wellbeing, healthy digestion, and improved maturing.

3. Matcha is a great device to improve your exercises since it's empowering and calming.

4. The excellent splendid green tea has even been found to forestall malignancy because the cancer prevention agents in the tea are so high, they help ward off resistant system trespassers known as free radicals.

5. Matcha is multiple times higher in chlorophyll than regular tea. Chlorophyll is the green shade found in plants that can help give you clear skin, ensure your blood and heart, and help forestall joint inflammation.

6. One glass of matcha green tea is equivalent to the measure of nourishment found in 10 cups of ordinary tea.

7. The matcha green tea raises digestion, give a long stream of vitality versus an accident you get with espresso, and potentially help with weight the executives. Matcha isn't a substitution for an unhealthy diet. However, it is a lot more astute, an all-encompassing method to raise your digestion and additional vitality.

8. Matcha additionally brings nervousness due to the high, crude measures of L-theanine found in matcha. L-theanine is an amino corrosive that advances a condition of unwinding and is the explanation standard green tea is thought of as a quieting drink.

9. Matcha just contains 35 milligrams of caffeine for each teaspoon, which is very nearly a third, not precisely some ordinary dark espresso.

Sounds quite astonishing for a tea, isn't that so? That is because matcha, similar to all plant-based foods, has stimulating properties that make it uncommon in its light. Recollect that matcha is not a handy solution enchantment pill to consummate wellbeing, yet it sure beats out different teas and is a superior, less-handled choice.

Appreciate Matcha Green Tea

Customary use: Matcha can be delighted. Similarly, you would utilize regular green tea, and you simply need to blend it a piece in an unexpected way. Heat a cup and a portion of water, pour it in your preferred tea mug, and let it sit for 3-5 minutes, at that point rush in 1/2 teaspoon of matcha green tea powder. You'll see it begins to froth a piece, and this is normal. You can likewise include a little non-dairy milk if you like, which will give it a creamier flavor. Or on the other hand, mix everything in your blender to make it frothier like bistro style drinks.

Different utilizations: Matcha is additionally astonishing in a green smoothie. You can utilize it to supplant your typical green superfood powder with a squeeze, or simply use it in some other customary smoothie. Since it's so high in nourishment, you needn't bother with a great deal of it to get the medical advantages. A half to an entire teaspoon is the bounty.

You can likewise utilize matcha in vitality nibbles, veggie lover ice cream, truffles, and even prepare brownies and cupcakes. Or then again, keep things basic and mix it with some ice and non-dairy milk to make a frosted matcha latte.

Matcha and What to Look for:

It's significant not to purchase only any old brand of matcha tea. Numerous brands advertise matcha tea that isn't correct matcha. The better brands will be somewhat pricier than modest forms you find at the market, and this demonstrates their higher caliber. Check the mark on all matcha you purchase. It should just incorporate 100 % matcha green tea leaves and ideally be natural and formal evaluation, which demonstrates it's created in the equivalent, insignificantly handling method of green tea expended in Japan and will guarantee it contains no pesticides.

The shading ought to likewise be a brilliant green, not a sloppy greenish-earthy colored shading, which demonstrates it's been all the more vigorously prepared or is a less expensive assortment of matcha.

Most matcha is sold in 2-4 ounce holders and ranges somewhere in the range of $15.00-$50.00 per compartment. These are unquestionably not modest but rather will last at any rate three months if you utilize a half teaspoon for each day.

A diet that underlines dim chocolate, red wine, kale, berries, and espresso? It either seems like the ideal street to health and weight loss, or unrealistic. However, pause, it shows signs of improvement: According to the creators of the Sirtfood Diet, these and other alleged "sirtfoods" are indicated to enact the systems constrained by your body's regular "thin qualities" to assist you with consuming fat and get in shape.

CHAPTER FOUR

A SIMPLE WEEKLY GUIDE THAT FOLLOWS YOU DAY AFTER DAY

The one bit of pack you have to follow the Sirtfood Diet is a juicer to make the essential day by day green juices. While there's heaps of discussion about which juicers are ideal, we're not hugely hung up on that. Simply get one that you can manage. You'll likewise need to get some matcha green tea powder to add to your juices as it's a great fat-consuming sirtfood. Attempt Love Matcha Grade Green Tea Powder (£6.99 for 50g, from Amazon). Another option – even though not as ground-breaking – is to keep the powder separate from the juice and drink three cups of green tea every day.

Your meal planner

This diet depends on a two-phase, three-week plan. Week one is a concentrated seven-day program intended to launch weight loss. Weeks two and three are an upkeep plan designed for proceeded with weight loss (expect around 1-2lbs per week) and better wellbeing.

Pick your meal decisions from the rundown.

WEEK 1

Day 1 to 3 (1,000 calories for each day)

- Breakfast: Sirtfood green juice

- Mid-morning: Green juice

- Lunch: Green juice

- Dinner: Choice from underneath, in addition to 15–20g dim chocolate

Day 4 to 7 (1,500 calories for every day)

Plan as above, however you drop one of the days by day green squeezes and supplant it with a second every day meal – either breakfast or lunch from the rundown.

WEEKS 2 AND 3

Every day ought to include:

- 3 x sirtfood primary meals
- 1 sirtfood green juice
- 2 snacks, browse a little bunch of pecans, strawberries or blueberries or an apple

Breakfasts

- Green juice
- Sirtfood omelet – with bacon, parsley, chicory
- Greek yogurt – with 10g ground dull chocolate, slashed pecans and blended berries
- Spiced fried eggs – with stew and turmeric

Lunches

- Baked cod with sautéed greens

- Vegetable and kidney bean stew with heated potato

- Waldorf plate of mixed greens with red onion, celery, apples, and pecans

- Baked chicken bosom with pecan and parsley pesto and red onion plate of mixed greens

Dinners

- Prawn pan sear with buckwheat noodles

- Chicken bosom with tomato and bean stew salsa

- Salmon filet with chicory, rocket and celery serving of mixed greens

- Beef with red wine, onion rings, and herb simmered potatoes

- Tuscan bean stew

Sirtfood green juice (Serves 1)

Ingredients

- Two huge bunches (75g) kale

- Huge bunch (30g) rocket

- Small bunch (5g) level leaf parsley

- 2–3 huge stems (150g) green celery – including leaves

- A large portion of a green apple

- Juice of half lemon and half tsp. Matcha.

To make:

1.   Juice all the ingredients except for the green tea. At that point, blend a limited quantity of juice in a glass with the matcha and mix overwhelmingly with a fork. At that point, including the remainder of the juice to the glass and blend once more.

2.   You can make up the entirety of your juices for the day in one group in the first part of the day and refrigerate until required.

Prawn Stir-fry with Noodles (Serves 1)

Ingredients
- 150g shelled crude prawns

- 2 tsp. soy sauce

- 2 tsp. additional virgin olive oil

- 75g soba (buckwheat noodles)

- One cleaved garlic clove

- 1 tsp. finely cleaved new ginger

- 20g red onions - cut

- 40g celery, cut

- 75g green beans – cleaved

- 50g cleaved kale

- 100ml chicken stock.

To make:

1.   Cook the prawns in a hot skillet with 1tsp of the soy and one tsp. of the oil for 2 minutes and put to the other side. Cook the noodles as coordinated on the bundle. Channel and put in a safe spot.

2.   Meanwhile, fry flavors and veg in the rest of the oil over medium-high heat for 2–3 minutes. Add the stock and bring to the bubble, at that point stew for a moment or two, until the vegetables are cooked yet at the same time crunchy.

3.   Add the prawns and noodles to the skillet, take back to the bubble. Expel from the heat and serve.

Hamburger with red wine, onion rings, and herb simmered potatoes (serves 1)

Ingredients

- 100g potatoes - stripped and cut into 2cm lumps

- 1 tsp. additional virgin olive oil

- 5g parsley - finely hacked

- 50g red onion-cut into rings

- 50g cut kale

- 1 garlic clove - finely hacked

- 150g meat steak

- 40ml red wine

- 150ml meat stock

- 1 tsp. tomato purée

- 1 tsp. Cornflour - broke up in 1 tsp. water

To make:

1.   Heat the stove to 220C/gas 7. Heat the potatoes for 5 minutes, at that point channel—a spot in a roasting tin with 1 tsp of the oil and dish for 35–45 minutes. Turn like clockwork. At the point when cooked, evacuate, sprinkle with the slashed parsley, and blend well.

2.	Fry onion in 1 tsp. of the oil over medium heat for 5–7 minutes, until pleasantly caramelized. Steam the kale for 2–3 minutes at that point channel. Fry the garlic delicately in 1⁄2 teaspoon of oil for 1 moment, until delicate, include the kale and fry for a further 1–2 minutes, until careful.

3.	Coat the meat with 1⁄2 a teaspoon of the oil and fry in a hot skillet over medium heat, as indicated by how you like it cooked. Expel from the dish and put aside to rest.

4.	Add the wine to the hot dish and lessen significantly, until sweet. Include the stock and tomato purée and bring to the bubble; at that point, add the cornflour glue to thicken a little at once. Serve hamburger with cook potatoes, kale, onion rings, and red wine sauce.

Tuscan bean stew (Serves 1)

Ingredients

- 1 tsp. additional virgin olive oil
- 50g red onion, finely cleaved 30g carrot, finely slashed 30g celery, finely hacked
- 1 garlic clove, finely cleaved
- 1 tsp. herbes de Provence 200ml vegetable stock
- 1 x 400g tin cleaved tomatoes 1 tsp. tomato purée
- 200g tinned blended beans
- 50g kale, cleaved
- 1 tsp. cleaved parsley
- 40g buckwheat to serve

To make:

1. Heat the oil and tenderly fry the onion, carrot, celery, garlic, and herbs, until the veg is delicate.

2. Add the stock, tomatoes, and tomato purée and bring it to the bubble. Include the beans and stew for 30 minutes.

Include the kale and cook for another 5–10 minutes until delicate, at that point, include the parsley.

3.   Cook the buckwheat as indicated by bundle instructions, channels, and serve.

At 1,200 calories, this veggie lover dinner plan sets you up to lose a sound 1 to 2 pounds for consistently and joins an arrangement of nutritious sustenance and balanced dinners to guarantee you're getting the enhancements you need each day. Whether or not you're a full-time veggie darling or scanning for strong vegan recipe considerations, this plant-based gala plan makes for seven days of healthy eating.

The best method to Meal Prep You Week of Meals:

1.   Make a gathering of the Vegan Pancakes to have for breakfast on Days 1, 5, and 7. Store the cooked hotcakes in a single layer in a water/air evidence holder and cement until arranged to eat; warm in the microwave.

2.   Cook a gathering of Basic Quinoa to have for lunch on Day 2 and dinner on Day 5.

3.   Make the Quinoa and Chia Oatmeal Mix and have on Day 4. Store the dry mix in an impervious holder for whatever length of time that month.

Day 1

Breakfast (296 calories)

- 2 Vegan Pancakes
- 1/4 cup blackberries
- 1 Tbsp. nutty spread

Mix nutty spread in with 1 tsp—warm water. Sprinkle over hotcakes.

A.M. Nibble (150 calories)

- 3/4 cup edamame units, arranged with a dash of salt

- 1 serving White Bean and Avocado Toast
- 1 cup cut cucumber

P.M. (30 calories)

- 1 little plum

Dinner (499 calories)

- 1 serving Falafel Salad with Lemon-Tahini Dressing

Day 2

Breakfast (262 calories)

- 1 serving Peanut Butter and Chia Berry Jam English Muffin

A.M. (100 calories)

- 1/2 cup edamame units, arranged with a pinch of salt

Lunch (360 calories)

- 4 cups White Bean and Veggie Salad

If you're taking this plate of blended greens to go, get it together in this helpful gala prep compartment, expressly made to keep your greens new and dressing separate until you're set up to eat.

Dinner (500 calories)

- 2 cups Black-Bean Quinoa Buddha Bowl

Day 3

Breakfast (266 calories)

- 1 serving Peanut Butter-Banana Toast

A.M. Goody (114 calories)

- 2 Tbsp. pumpkin seeds (pepitas)

Lunch (325 calories)

- 4 cups serving Green Salad with Edamame and Beets

P.M. Goody (62 calories)

- 2 cups air-popped popcorn

Dinner (446 calories)

- 1 1/2 cups Roasted Cauliflower and Potato Curry Soup

- 1/2 minimal whole wheat pita, toasted

- 1/3 cup hummus

Banquet Prep Tip: Save one serving of the Roasted Cauliflower and Potato Curry Soup in a watertight dinner prep holder for lunch on Day 4.

Day 4

Breakfast (296 calories)

- 1/3 cup Quinoa and Chia Oatmeal Mix cooked with 1/4 cups unsweetened soymilk

Banquet Prep Tip: Make the Quinoa and Chia Oatmeal Mix and store in a fixed shut compartment for whatever length of time that month.

A.M. Goody (30 calories)

- 1 little plum

Lunch (309 calories)

- 1 1/2 cups Roasted Cauliflower and Potato Curry Soup

- 1/2 minimal whole wheat pita, toasted

P.M. Goody (114 calories)

- 2 Tbsp. pumpkin seeds (pepitas)

Dinner (472 calories)

- 1 serving Stuffed Sweet Potato with Hummus Dressing

Day 5

Breakfast (296 calories)

- 2 Vegan Pancakes

- 1/4 cup blackberries

- 1 Tbsp. nutty spread

Mix nutty spread in with 1 tsp—warm water (or progressively, shifting, to scatter the nutty spread). Sprinkle over hotcakes.

Lunch (325 calories)

- 1 serving Veggie and Hummus Sandwich

P.M. Chomp (100 calories)

- 1/2 cup edamame units, arranged with a bit of salt

Dinner (487 calories)

- 1 cup Chickpea Curry
- 1 cup Basic Quinoa

Day 6

Breakfast (262 calories)

- 1 serving Peanut Butter and Chia Berry Jam English Muffin

A.M. (17 calories)

- 1/4 cup hummus
- 2 medium celery stems, cut into sticks

Lunch (308 calories)

- 1 serving Vegan Bistro Lunch Box
- 2 Tbsp. pumpkin seeds (pepitas)

Dinner (525 calories)

- 1 serving Thai Spaghetti Squash with Peanut Sauce
- 1 cup Vegan Thai Cucumber Salad

Day 7

Breakfast (296 calories)

- 2 Vegan Pancakes
- 1/4 cup blackberries
- 1 Tbsp. nutty spread

Mix nutty spread in with 1 tsp—warm water. Sprinkle over hotcakes.

A.M. Goody (62 calories)

- 1 medium orange

Lunch (325 calories)

- 4 cups serving Green Salad with Edamame and Beets

P.M. Goody (93 calories)

- 3 cups air-popped popcorn

Dinner (434 calories)

- 1 serving Rainbow Veggie Spring Roll Bowl

You Did It!

Well done on finishing this veggie darling weight decrease dinner plan. Perhaps you followed every single dinner and snack or possibly basically used it as an authoritative guide for developing a veggie sweetheart diet. Regardless, we believe you found this course of action fascinating, delightful, and edifying. Following a plant-based eating routine, a dinner plan is a sound method to get fit as a fiddle and keep it off.

Continue doing magnificent one of our other sound veggie darling dinner plans or vegetarian feast plans.

Alongside this fat-consuming impact, sirtfoods additionally have the novel capacity to -naturally control craving and increment muscle work – making them the ideal answer for accomplishing a healthy weight. In reality, their wellbeing boosting impacts are ground-breaking to the point that a few investigations have demonstrated them to be more compelling than physician recommended tranquilizes in forestalling incessant malady, with clear -benefits in diabetes, coronary illness, and - Alzheimer's sickness. No prominent surprise societies eating the most sirtfoods – including Japan and Italy – are the least fatty and most beneficial on the planet. What's more, that is the reason we've conceived a diet based around them.

The sirtfood list

Sirtfoods are on the whole promptly accessible and -accessible foods. The strongest ones include red wine, dim chocolate, dark espresso, kale, rocket, parsley, red onions, strawberries, pecans, additional virgin olive oil, curry flavors, green tea, blueberries, celery, bean stew, apples, and buckwheat.

What's the proof?

Trialing diet at a rec center in South West London, mainly to test and improve wellbeing. We were shocked by the outcomes. Members frequently lost 7lbs in seven days and saw increments in bulk, prosperity, and vitality. We anticipated that individuals should lose some weight yet never foreseen that it would be such a lot, nor that individuals would keep up or even add some muscle, which is exceptionally unordinary when dieting.

CHAPTER FIVE

TOP SIRTFOODS- 20 FOODS THAT ACTIVATE WEIGHT LOSS

These are the most elevated and evaluated 20 foods for a Sirtfood-rich diet, and how you can fuse them into your day by day meals

1.   Bird's eye stew - Also sold as Thai chilies, they're more potent than ordinary bean stews, and increasingly pressed with supplements. Use them to set off sweet or acrid recipes.

2.   Buckwheat - Technically a pseudo-grain: it's an organic product seed identified with rhubarb. Likewise accessible in noodle structure (as soba), yet ensure you're getting the without wheat rendition.

3.   Capers - if you're pondering, they're salted bloom buds. Sprinkle them over a plate of mixed greens or simmered cauliflower.

4.   Celery - The hearts and leaves are the most nutritious part, so don't discard them in case you're mixing up a shake.

5.   Cocoa - The flavonol-rich kind improves pulse, glucose control, and cholesterol. Search for a high level of cacao.

6.   Coffee - Drink it darksome proof milk can decrease the assimilation of sirtuin-actuating supplements.

7.   Extra virgin olive oil - The new virgin kind has more Sirt benefits, and an all the more fulfilling, peppery taste.

8.   Green tea or matcha - Add a cut of lemon to build retention of sirtuin-delivering supplements. Matcha is far and away superior; however, go Japanese, not Chinese, to stay away from potential lead sullying.

9.   Kale - Includes large measures of sirtuin-enacting supplements quercetin and kaempferol. Back rub it with olive

oil and lemon juice to serve it as a plate of mixed greens.

10.	Lovage - It's a herb. Become your on a windowsill, and toss it into sautés.

11.	Medjool dates - They're a weighty 66% sugar; however - with some restraint - don't raise glucose levels and have been connected to bring traces of diabetes and coronary illness.

12.	Parsley - More than only a trimming – it's high in apigenin. Toss it into a smoothie or juice for the full advantage.

13.	Chicory - Red is ideal, however yellow works fine. Toss it in a plate of mixed greens.

14.	Red onion - The red assortment's better for you, and sufficiently sweet to eat crude. Hack it and add to a serving of mixed greens, or eat it with a burger.

15.	Red wine - You've known about resveratrol: the uplifting news is, it's heat stable, so you can get profits by cooking with it (just as glugging it straight). Pinot noir has the most noteworthy substance.

16.	Rocket - One of the least meddled with serving of mixed greens accessible. Sprinkle it with olive oil.

17.   Soy - Soybeans and miso are high in sirtuin activators. Remember it for sautés.

18.   Strawberries - Though they're sweet, they just contain 1tsp of sugar per 100g – and look into recommends they improve your body's capacity to deal with delicious carbs.

19.   Turmeric - Evidence proposes the curcumin in it has against malignancy properties. It's hard for the body to acclimatize alone; however, cooking it in fluid and including fat and dark pepper expands retention.

20.   Walnuts - High in fat and calories, however, settled in decreasing metabolic sickness. Crush them up with parsley for sirt-enhanced pesto.

These are the main twenty Sirtfoods and the establishment of the Sirtfood Diet. Sirtfoods are plant foods wealthy in explicit polyphenols that actuate our sirtuin qualities. Eating them turns on a reusing procedure in our phones, getting out all the messiness and waste that develops with age and regularly causes sick wellbeing. To fuel this reusing procedure, our cells tap into our fat stores.

The result of this is restored cells, wellbeing, and vitality, and weight loss.

- Sirtuins are ace metabolic controllers that control our capacity to consume fat and remain healthy

- Sirtuins go about as vitality sensors inside our cells and are enacted when a lack of vitality is distinguished

- Fasting and exercise both enact our sirtuin qualities however these can be difficult to continue with and may have disadvantages

By eating a diet wealthy in the leading 20 Sirtfoods, you can emulate the impacts of fasting and practice and accomplish a more advantageous body

Sirtfood Diet Green Juice

The Sirtfood Diet green juice is a significant piece of the Sirtfood Diet. It is incorporated among the recipes remembered for the Best Sirtfood Recipes page, so we figured it is useful to combine the recipe independently here. Regardless of whether you have no aim of following the diet, the juice is stuffed loaded with supplements and would be a great expansion to a standard diet. One significant thing to note: We have looked into cautiously, and you need to make this in a juicer, NOT a blender (or a Nutribullet or food processor, or whatever else other than a juicer). We have given the two different ways a shot and can report that the mixed form is a fearful tasting slop, the squeezed rendition is a sensibly pleasant tasting juice!

The Sirtfood Diet green juice will keep for as long as three days in the ice chest, so it's well worth making up a significant clump to spare time. We, as a rule, make the juices up the prior night to spare time in the mornings. This Sirtfood Diet green juice is pressed with supplement rich Sirtfoods, great for anybody needing somewhat of a wellbeing lift and basic for anybody following the Sirtfood Diet.

Ingredients

- 75g kale

- 30g rocket

- 5g parsley

- 2 celery sticks

- ½ green apple

- 1cm ginger

- Juice of ½ lemon

- ½ teaspoon matcha green tea

Method

1.   Juice all the ingredients separated from the lemon and the matcha green tea.

2.   Squeeze the lemon juice into the green squeeze by hand.

3.   Pour a modest quantity of green juice into a glass and mix it in the matcha. Include the remainder of the green juice into the glass and mix once more.

4.   Drink straight away or put something aside for some other time.

Sirtfoods with Other Foods

We realize that Sirtfoods and some different foods are beneficial for us, regardless of whether its veggies like broccoli or tomatoes, flavors like turmeric, or refreshments like green tea. The explanation these – and numerous other plant foods – are beneficial for us, is principal to the bio-dynamic plant mixes they contain. For the healthfully clever, we may be considering sulforaphane from broccoli, lycopene from tomatoes, curcumin from turmeric, and catechins from green tea. All the subject of broad logical research that goes far to clarifying exactly why these foods are so useful for our wellbeing.

Yet rather than simply eating those individual foods, on a par with they, imagine a scenario where blending certain foods – and hence their supplements – together at meals conveyed a considerably greater wellbeing help. Imagine a scenario where we could create collaborations between supplements in various foods that intensify their medical advantages. It's another thought, and here are the best five of instances of how foods (and you will perceive the Sirtfoods in this rundown) can include for greatest impact.

1. Green tea + lemon: Green tea consumers can expect various medical advantages given that devouring this prized drink is connected with less malignancy, coronary illness, diabetes, and osteoporosis. These medical advantages can be clarified by its remarkable substance of plant mixes called catechins, and particularly a sort called epigallocatechin gallate (EGCG). Including a crush of lemon juice to your green tea, which is plentiful in nutrient C, serves to fundamentally build the measure of catechins that get retained into the body.

2. Tomato sauce + additional virgin olive oil: Lycopene is the carotenoid answerable for the dark red shade of tomatoes, and its utilization is connected with a decreased danger of specific malignant growths (most remarkably malignant growth of the prostate), cardiovascular malady, osteoporosis, and in any event, shielding the skin from the harming impacts of the sun. The principal thing to think about lycopene is that cooking and handling tomatoes significantly build the measure of lycopene that the body can retain. The second is

that the nearness of fat further builds lycopene ingestion. So collaborating your tomato-based dishes with a liberal shower of additional virgin olive oil bodes well.

3. Turmeric + dark pepper: Turmeric, the splendid yellow flavor ever-present in customary Indian cooking, is the subject of extreme logical examination for its enemy of malignant growth properties, it's the capability to lessen inflammation in the body, and in any event, for fighting off dementia. This is accepted to be basically because of its dynamic constituent curcumin. In any case, the issue with curcumin is that it is ineffectively consumed by the body. Nonetheless, including dark pepper expands its assimilation, making them the ideal flavor twofold act. Cooking turmeric in fluid, and including fat, further assists with curcumin retention.

4. Broccoli + mustard: it's an obvious fact that broccoli is beneficial for us, with benefits including diminishing malignancy chance. Broccoli's fundamental malignancy preventive ingredient is sulforaphane. This is shaped when we eat broccoli by the activity of a catalyst found in broccoli

called myrosinase. Notwithstanding, cooking broccoli – particularly over-cooking it – starts to obliterate the myrosinase compound, lessening the measure of sulforaphane that can be made. In case we're not cautious, we can cook the advantages directly out of broccoli. Nonetheless, for the individuals who like their broccoli all around cooked (as opposed to daintily steamed for 2 to 4 minutes), including other characteristic wellsprings of myrosinase, for example, from mustard or horseradish, implies that sulforaphane can even now be made.

5. A plate of mixed greens + avocado: Green verdant vegetables, for example, kale, spinach, and watercress are stuffed loaded with wellbeing advancing carotenoids, for example, invulnerable reinforcing beta-carotene and eye-accommodating lutein. However, when eaten crudely, as servings of mixed greens, these carotenoids are progressively hard to ingest. Yet, the option of some fat can truly help with that and including avocado, wealthy in monounsaturated fat, to a plate of mixed greens, has been appeared to expand the number of carotenoids that can be consumed drastically.

Appreciate the Sirtfoods with options and receive the additional wellbeing rewards.

Sirtfood - What are Medjool Dates?

Medjool dates are a kind of organic tree product that starts in the Middle East and North Africa, yet they can be developed with some achievement in various desert-like locales around the globe. Dates all in all make up a significant piece of Middle Eastern food, yet Medjools especially are prized for their enormous size, their sweet taste, and their succulent tissue in any event, when dried. They are regularly delighted in all alone as a tidbit or as a seasoning component inside a bigger meal or prepared sweet.

The Difference from Other Sorts of Dates

There are lots of assortments of dates. However, all offer some fundamental attributes. They develop on date palm trees, for example, and are local to hot, bone-dry atmospheres. Their organic product can be eaten new; however, it is all the more normally dried, which protracts its life expectancy and forestalls early waste. Medjool dates are generally viewed as the "best" assortment of dates. They are positively the biggest and are generally additionally the most costly to purchase. Numerous purchasers accept that they have the most extravagant flavor also.

Medjools are frequently casually known as the "lord of dates," the "precious stone of dates," or the "cream of dates" regarding their raised position. They are what is known as a "delicate" date. The organic products are normally arranged as delicate, dry, or semi-dry concerning their surface and taste. Delicate dates are typically viewed as the most lovely to a limited extent as a result of how much harder they are to develop, just as the amount progressively defenseless they are to lose by winged animals and bugs.

Taste Basics of Medjool Dates

The vast majority portray Medjool dates as having a rich, practically caramel-like taste, and notices of nectar and cinnamon are likewise normal. They are normally served dried, yet this drying normally happens much of the time. The most customary approach to plan dates of any sort is to permit them to age and afterward sundry while still associated with the tree. When picked at the correct time, Medjools need no extra treatment or care before serving.

Wholesome Profile

Medjool dates just contain around 66 calories each. They are a decent wellspring of fiber and contain significant levels of basic minerals, potassium, magnesium, copper, and manganese. Most contain a lot of organic product sugar. However, this can make them a decent option, in contrast, to progressively caloric treats. In the Middle East, where they develop wild, they are a well-known food for roaming voyagers as they give a great deal of vitality and invigorating supplements with the additional advantage of being promptly accessible.

Step by Step Instructions to Enjoy Medjool Dates

Probably the most straightforward approach to appreciate Medjool dates is to eat them all alone, either as an autonomous bite or close by other finger foods like hard cheeses, saltines, and dried up bread. The dates do contain a pit; however, it is large and, for the most part, simple to expel.

The organic product's huge size likewise loans well to stuffing once the pit has been evacuated. Pecans, almonds, and honeycomb are a portion of the more customary things that cooks can put inside, yet there is a great deal of space for creativity. A few people put different organic products, little bits of chocolate, or exquisite meats into the pit to create a stand-out taste.

Use in Cooking

Medjool dates additionally feature in various recipes. Numerous North African stews call for cut Medjools, for example, and they are normally blended in with yogurt for breakfast in nations like Iraq and Iran. They add pleasantness to various cooked meat dishes and can likewise be joined into the hitter of a wide range of bread and prepared products.

Where They Grow

Date palms that offer ascent to Medjool organic products are accepted to be indigenous toward the North African coast and Arabic Peninsula. Fossil proof proposes that the organic products were delighted in by old individuals in nations as far separated as Saudi Arabia and Morocco, and the land between these nations remains the essential developing zone. Numerous California ranchers have had some karma developing the trees, however, as have a few people in Australia. They are regularly a lot harder to develop than other date assortments in light of how touchy the organic products are to air quality and soil dampness. They regularly take a colossal measure of work to develop on request, which is a piece of the explanation behind their generally significant expense.

Development at Home

The essential approach to growing a Medjool date palm is to plant a pit and sit tight for it to grow. However, this is likewise the most tedious and conceivably disappointing method. It can take as long as 20 years for a green pit to yield a tree that proves to be fruitful. Home cultivators needing to take a stab at developing Medjools are normally better served by buying set up plants from nurseries or nearby merchants or joining branches from existing palms onto new plants. Trees normally need a great deal of care, just as close consideration regarding daylight and soil quality, to flourish. A few cultivators have had achievements developing the plants in indoor nurseries. However, the best organic products will, in general, originate from trees presented to increasingly common outside settings.

CHAPTER SIX

HOW TO FOLLOW THE SIRTFOOD DIET

These are the features of the Sirtfood Diet—however, there's more to it than eating chocolate, drinking wine, and shedding pounds. The idea driving the diet is that you eat certain foods that will turn on your "thin quality," which triggers a course of responses that at last lead to "weight loss and improved protection from an ailment," as portrayed in the book The Sirtfood Diet.

The diet purportedly helped vocalist Adele lose 50 lb. Sounds unrealistic? Possibly, perhaps not. We should investigate this chocolate-and-wine diet and check whether the science backs up its "clinically demonstrated" routine.

The Sirtfood Diet was begun by a couple of nutritionists in England. Their idea is that when you cut calories or quick, your body's phones call for vitality, which initiates the "thin quality." This quality (a gathering of qualities called sirtuins) triggers a series of responses. For one, the body switches into "endurance mode," stopping its typical development forms. Thus, it quits putting away fat and starts consuming it. What's more, presto, weight loss.

The issue with this fasting procedure is that it can prompt craving, just as crabbiness, exhaustion, and muscle loss.

Here's the place the dull chocolate and red wine come in. The authors of the diet say that specific foods—"sirtfoods"— are particularly wealthy in explicit polyphenols that initiate the equivalent sirtuin qualities that fasting triggers. In this way, by eating these foods, you enact the sirtuin (thin) qualities, which hence consume fat so you get thinner—all without the reaction of craving, as per the diet's originators.

In any case, that is not all: Sirtuins additionally seem to diminish inflammation and fix cell harm, making you more beneficial.

Eminent sirtfoods include:

Buckwheat

Celery

Cocoa

Espresso

Additional virgin olive oil

Green tea (matcha)

Kale

Lovage

Medjool dates

Parsley

Red onion

Red wine

Soy

Strawberries

Turmeric

Pecans

What's the plan?

The objective of the main week of the 3-week Sirtfood Diet is to lose 7 lb. This is finished by eating and drinking an aggregate of just 1,000 calories of just sirtfoods a day for the initial three days. The majority of these calories are expended in green squeeze (an invention made of kale, arugula, parsley, celery, green apple, lemon juice, and matcha green tea).

For the following four days, you eat and drink what could be compared to around 1,500 calories for each day in sirtfoods. As indicated by the diet's creators, individuals who follow this program don't get especially ravenous.

The accompanying two weeks of the diet is the support phase, in which you should keep on consistently get more fit. During this phase, you eat three sirtfood-rich meals and one green juice for every day, with no calorie limitations.

After this 3-week compressed lesson, you keep up your (foreseen) astounding weight loss and recently discovered wellbeing by normally incorporating sirtfoods in your meals and chugging the green squeeze each day.

How Can It Work?

As we referenced above, diet depends on this idea of "thin" sirtuin qualities. Things being what they are, what right? In warm-blooded creatures, the sirtuin qualities produce a gathering of seven proteins that were at first appeared to slow maturing in yeast. These proteins were additionally found to build a life span in mice. Besides, the sirtuin proteins can be actuated by calorie limitation and by polyphenols. The polyphenol that has been most researched in such manner is resveratrol, the compound found in red wine and dim chocolate.

Thus, in principle, this diet should work. Lower your calories and eat sirtfoods (which are rich in polyphenols), and—bam! — The sirtuins will kick in and begin consuming fat. Surely, analysts have indicated that the enactment of the Sirt1 (sirtuin

1) compound consumes fat (white fat tissue) in mouse fat cells just as in live mice.

That is great for rotund mice. In any case, up until now, the fat-consuming impact hasn't been demonstrated in people, despite research that explicitly explored this inquiry. In one little investigation in people, for example, resveratrol and caloric limitation did for sure increment serum convergences of Sirt1. However, just the caloric limitation was liable for diminishing individuals' midsection size and bringing lipid levels.

In any case, if initiating sirtuins could consume fat and diminish weight in people, it would be an enormous turn of events. Keeping that in mind, various scientists and pharmaceutical organizations are caught up with building up a sirtuin-activating medication that could do only that.

Eating a diet that incorporates a ton of "sirtfoods"— that is, foods high in cell reinforcement, mitigating polyphenols—and cutting calories is a genuinely healthy and likely useful activity, nutritionists' state. However, this specific diet, particularly during the prohibitive first week, doesn't seem to give enough calories or a wide enough assortment of foods to make it practical. There's nothing amiss with a chomp of chocolate and a taste of a wine once in a while.

CHAPTER SEVEN

PHASES OF SIRTFOOD DIET

Sirtfoods are foods that initiate SIRT1 qualities. Sirtfoods are predominantly plant-based foods that contain incredible phytonutrients (plant supplements). These enact the sirtuin-actuating biochemicals, which in any case, just get initiated in light of pressure like fasting or working out.

At the point when you devour these Sirtfoods, your body emulates the pressure reaction without you having to, in reality, quick or exercise. Henceforth, you consume calories/fat without losing bulk, without fasting, and without doing energetic activities. In the accompanying segment, we will investigate the foods you can eat on the Sirtfood diet.

The Sirtfood Diet is so fascinated by the capability of Sirtfoods. They created a diet based around amplifying Sirtfood consumption and mellow calorie limitation. They, at that point, tried this diet on members from a selective London rec center and were astonished by their discoveries. Rec center individuals lost a normal of 7lbs in the initial seven days, despite not expanding their degrees of activity. Not exclusively did the members lose a generous measure of weight. However, they additionally picked up muscle (as a rule the inverse happens when dieting) and detailed noteworthy enhancements in general wellbeing and prosperity.

So, How Does the Sirtfood Diet Work?
The diet is part of 2 phases. Phase 1: the seven day 'hyper success phase', which joins a Sirtfood-rich diet with moderate

calorie limitation, and Phase 2: the 14-day' upkeep phase,' where you combine your weight loss without confining calories.

Phase 1 of the Sirtfood Diet

During the initial three days, calorie admission is confined to 1,000 calories (along these lines, still more than on a 5:2 fasting day). The diet comprises of 3 Sirtfood-rich green juices and 1 Sirtfood-rich meal and two squares of dim chocolate.

During the staying four days, calorie admission is expanded to 1, 500 calories, and every day the diet includes 2 Sirtfood-rich green juices and 2 Sirtfood-rich meals.

During the first phase, you are not permitted to drink any liquor. However, you can drink water, tea, espresso, and green tea unreservedly.

Phase 2 of the Sirtfood Diet

Phase 2 doesn't concentrate on calorie limitation. Every day includes 3 Sirtfood-rich meals and one green juice, in addition to the choice of 1 or 2 Sirtfood chomp snacks, whenever required.

In phase 2, you are permitted to drink red wine, yet with some restraint (the suggestion is 2-3 glasses of red wine every week), just as water, tea, espresso, and green tea.

What are the Sirtfood Diet and accomplishes it truly work? Is there an eating plan for the sirtfood diet?

Indeed, there is a useful diagram mentioning to you about what you can eat every day and when. The book has all the recipes you will require for the initial three weeks. There is a meat/fish choice and a veggie lover/vegetarian choice for consistently. Practically all the recipes are without gluten, and there are sans dairy alternatives consistently, meaning this is a diet that will work for a great many people.

What are the Sirtfood Diet and accomplishes it truly work? What occurs after you have completed the sirtfood diet?

The Sirtfood Diet isn't intended to be an erratic 'diet' but instead a lifestyle. You are supported, when you've finished the initial three weeks, to keep eating a diet rich in Sirtfoods and to keep drinking your day by day green juice. Since propelling their unique book, the writers of The Sirtfood Diet have proceeded to discharge The Sirtfood Diet Recipe Book, with recipes for parts more Sirtfood-rich fundamental meals, just as recipes for options in contrast to the green juice and more indications and tips for following the Sirtfood Diet. There are even a few recipes for Sirtfood treats! The creators of The Sirtfood Diet recommend that Phases 1 and 2 can be repeated as and when essential for a wellbeing help, or if things have gone somewhat off course.

Phase 1: 7 Pounds in Seven Days

Welcome to Phase 1 of the Sirtfood Diet. This is the hyper-achievement phase, where you will step toward accomplishing a slimmer and less fatty body. Follow our straightforward bit by bit instructions and utilize the delightful recipes accommodated you. Notwithstanding our standard seven-day plan, we likewise have a sans meat adaptation, which is appropriate for the two veggie lovers and vegetarians. Don't hesitate to go with whichever one you like.

What's in store?

During Phase 1, you will receive the full rewards of our clinically demonstrated method for shedding 7 pounds in seven days. However, recall this incorporates muscle gain, so don't get hung up absolutely with the numbers on the scales. N or should you start gauging yourself day by day. We regularly observe the scales flinch up over the most recent couple of days of Phase 1 because of muscle gain, while waistlines keep on contracting. That is the reason we need you to take a gander at the scales, however not be controlled by the. Look at what you look like in the mirror, how your garments are fitting, or whether you have to move an indent on your belt. These are largely great markers of the m metal significant changes in your body composition.

Be aware of different changes as well, for example, in your

feeling of well-being, your vitality levels, and how clear your skin looks. You can even get estimations of your general cardiovascular and metabolic wellbeing performed at your nearby drug store to s changes in things like your circulatory strain, glucose levels, and blood fats, for example, cholesterol and triglycerides. Keep in mind, weight loss aside, the presentation of Sirtfoods into your diet is an enormous advance in making your cells matter and progressively impervious to sickness, setting you up for a lifetime of remarkable wellbeing.

Step by Step Instructions to Follow Phase 1

To make Phase 1 as plain cruising as could reasonably be expected, we'll manage you through the total seven-day plan each day in turn, including the Sirtfood grape juice and simple-to-follow, tasty recipes each progression of the way.

Phase 1 of the Sirtfood Diet depends on two particular stages:

Days 1 to 3 are the most serious, and during this period you can eat up to a limit of 1,000 calories every day, comprising of:

- 3 x Sirtfood grape juices

- 1 x primary meal

Days 4 to 7 will s your food consumption increment to the furthest reaches of 1,500 calories every day, comprising of:

- 2 x Sirtfood grape juices

- 2 x fundamental meals

There are not many standards for following the diet. Eventually, it's tied in with placing it into your way of life and around day-to-day living for delayed achievement. However, here are a couple of basic yet enormous effect tips for accomplishing the best result:

1. Get a Good Juicer: Juicing is a basic piece of the Sirtfood Diet, and a juicer is probably the best venture you will make for your wellbeing. While spending plan ought to be the

deciding component, a few juicers are progressively powerful at removing the juice from green verdant vegetables and herbs, with the Breville brand being among the best of the accessible juicers we have attempted.

2. Arrangement Is Key: From the abundance off the back, we have made them clear: the individuals who planned ahead of time were the best. Get acquainted with the ingredients and recipes and stock up on what you need. With everything sorted out and prepared, you'll be surprised at how simple the entire procedure is.

3. Spare Time: If you are tight for time, get ready cunningly. Meals can be made the prior night. Juices can be made in mass and kept in the cooler for as long as three days (or longer in, the cooler) before their degrees of sirt in-actuating supplements begin to drop. Simply shield it from light, and possibly include the matcha when you are prepared to devour it.

4. Eat Early: It is smarter to eat prior in the day, and meals

and juices ought to in a perfect world not be expended later than 7 p.m; at the end of the day the diet is intended to work with your way of life, and late eaters despite everything receive a great reward.

5. Space out the Juices: To improve retention of the green juices, they ought to be expended in any event an hour prior or two hours after a meal and spread out for the duration of the day, as opposed to having them excessively near one another.

6. Eat until Satisfied: Sirtfoods can effectively affect craving, and a few people will be full before completing their meals. Tune in to your body and eat until you are fulfilled as opposed to compelling all the food down.

7. Appreciate the Journey: Don't get made up for lost time with the ultimate objective; rather, remain aware of the excursion. This diet is tied in with praising food in the entirety of its marvel for its medical advantages, however similarly for the joy and delight, it brings. Research shows that when we

keep our brains concentrated on the way rather than the last goal, we are considerably more liable to succeed.

What to Drink

As well as the suggested everyday servings of green juices, you can expend different liquids fry all through Phase 1. These ought to be no caloric beverages, ideally plain water, dark espresso, and green tea. If your standard al preference is for dark or home areas, fallowed to incorporate these too. Sodas and natural product juices are abandoned. Rather, if you w insect to jazz things up, take a stab at adding some cut strawberries to in any case or shimmering water to make your Sirtfood-injected wellbeing drink. Unit in the cooler for a few hours, and you'll have an agreeably invigorating option in contrast to soda pops and squeezes.

One thing to be aware of is that we don't prescribe abrupt changes to your standard al espresso utilization. Caffeine withdrawal indications can make you f lousy for two or three days; similarly, huge increments can be unsavory for those especially delicate with the impacts of caffeine. We additionally suggest that espresso be tanked dark, without including milk, since certain analysts have discovered that the option of m1 kind can lessen the ingestion of the

Helpful sirtuin-initiating supplements. The equivalent has been found for green tea, however, including some lemon squeeze expands the assimilation of its three sirtuin-actuating supplements.

Do recall this is the hyper-achievement phase, and keeping in mind that you ought to be supported by the way that it is for one week in particular, you should be more trained. For this, we incorporate liquor, like red wine, yet just as a cooking ingredient.

The Sirtfood Green Juice

The green juice is a fundamental piece of Phase 1 of the Sirtfood Diet. All the ingredients are amazing. Sirtfoods, and in every juice, you get a strong mixed drink of regular compounds, for example, apigenin, kaempferol, luteolin, quercetin, and E G C G that cooperate in turning on your sirtuin qualities and advancing fat loss. To that, we've included lemon, as its characteristic corrosiveness has been appeared to secure, settle, and increment the retention of the beverage's sirtuin-enacting supplements. We've additionally included a bit of apple and ginger for taste. Both of these are, in this way, discretionary. Ind, numerous individuals and that once they are acquainted with the flavor of the juice, they forget about the apple inside and out.

Sirtfood Green Juice (Serves 1)

- 2 huge bunches (around 21/2 ounces or 75g) kale

- A huge bunch (1 ounce or 30g) arugula

- An exceptionally little bunch (around 1/4 ounce or 5g) at-leaf parsley

- 2 to 3 huge celery stems (51/2 ounces or 150g), including leaves

- 1/2-to 1-inch (1 to 2.5 cm) bit of new ginger

- Juice of 1/2 lemon

- 1/2 level teaspoon coordinate a powder

Days 1 to 3 of Phase 1: added uniquely to the initial two juices of the day;

Days 4 to 7 of Phase 1: added to the two juices

Note that while in our pilot preliminary, all amounts were weighed out precisely as recorded, our experience is that bunch estimates work very well. They better tailor the supplement amount to a person's body size. Bigger people will, in general, have bigger hands and, in this manner, get a relatively higher measure of Sirtfood supplements to coordinate their body size and the other way around for littler individuals.

• Mix the grapes (kale, arugula, and parsley) and juice them. We find that juicers can truly vary in their proficiency at squeezing verdant vegetables, and you may need to re-juice the remainders before proceeding onward to different ingredients. The objective is to wind up with around two liquid ounces or near 1/4 cup (50m l) of juice from the greens.

• Now squeeze the celery, apple, and ginger.

• You can put   the lemon and put it through the juicer also, yet we think that its a lot simpler to just crush the lemon by hand into the juice. By this stage, you ought to have around 1 cup (250m l) of juice altogether, maybe somewhat more.

• It is just when the juice is made and prepared to serve that you include the matcha. Pour a modest quantity of the juice into a glass. At that point, include the matcha and mix overwhelmingly with a fork or teaspoon. We just use matcha in the initial two beverages of the day since it contains moderate measures of caffeine (a similar substance as a typical cup of tea). For individuals not accustomed to it, it may keep them alert whenever alcoholic late.

• Once the matcha is disintegrated, include the rest of the juice. Give it a last mix, ad your juice is prepared to drink. Don't hesitate to top up with plain water, as indicated by taste.

Phase 2: Maintenance

Congrats on finishing Phase 1 of the Sirtfood Diet! As of now, you ought to be seeing great outcomes with fat loss and are looking slimmer and increasingly conditioned, yet feeling renewed and reenergized. All in all, what now?

Having seen these frequently striking changes ourselves firsthand, we know the amount you'll w subterranean insect to safeguard each one of those advantages, yet observe far and away superior outcomes. Sirtfoods are intended to be eaten forever. The inquiry is the way you adjust what you have been doing in Phase 1 into your typical dietary daily practice. That is actually what provoked us to create a follow - up fourth-day upkeep plan intended to assist you with making the change from Phase 1 to your progressively ordinary dietary daily practice and, in this way, help support and further broaden the advantages of the Sirtfood Diet.

What's in store?
During Phase 2, you will unite your weight-loss results and keep on consistently lose weight.

Recall that the one striking thing we have found with the Sirtfood Diet is that most or the entirety of the weight that individuals lose is from fat and that numerous put on some muscle. So we w subterranean insect to remind you again not to pass judgment on your advancement absolutely by the numbers on the scale. Glance in the mirror to check whether you are looking less fatty and increasingly conditioned, perceive how your garments are fitting, and slurp up the commendations that you will get from others.

Recall excessively that similarly, as the weight loss will proceed, the medical advantages will develop. By following the fourteen-day support plan, you're truly beginning to set out the establishments for an eventual fate of long-lasting wellbeing.

Step by Step Instructions to Follow Phase 2

The way to achievement in this phase is to continue pressing your diet loaded with Sirtfoods. To make it as simple as could be expected under the circumstances, we've assembled a seven-day menu plan for you to follow, including delightful family-accommodating recipes, with every day pressed to the rafters with Sirtfoods (however observe page 149 for guidance in regards to children). All you n to do is repeat the seven-day plan twice to finish the fourth day of Phase 2.

On every one of the fourth days, your diet will comprise of:

• 3 x adjusted Sirtfood-rich meals

• 1 x Sirtfood grape juice

• 1 to 2 x discretionary Sirtfood chomp snacks

By and by, there are no unbending guidelines for when you need to expend these. Be adaptable and turn them around your day. Two basic general guidelines are:

• Have your grape juice either before anything else, in any event, thirty minutes before breakfast, or midmorning.

• Try your best to eat your night meal by 7 p.m.

Sizes of Portions

Our concentration during Phase 2 isn't on tallying calories. Over the drawn-out, this is not to earth or even fruitful methodology for the normal individual. Rather we're concentrating on reasonable bits, truly well-adjusted meals, and generally significant, topping off on Sirtfoods so you can keep on profiting by their fat-consuming and wellbeing advancing impacts.

We have additionally built the meals in the plan to make them satisfying, which will help you f full for more. That, joined with the common hunger managing impacts of Sirtfoods, implies that you won't go through the following fourth days feeling hungry, however rather charmingly fulfilled, well took care of, and all-around fed.

Similarly, as in Phase 1, make sure to tune in to your body and be guided by your hunger. If you get ready meals as indicated by our instructions and discover you are serenely full before you've completed a meal, at that point, it's impeccably ne to quit eating!

What to Drink

You will keep on including one green squeeze every day all through Phase 2. This is to keep you beat up with significant levels of Sirtfoods.

Similarly, as in Phase 1, you can devour different liquids unreservedly all through Phase 2.

Our favored beverages for you to incorporate stay plain water, custom made enhanced water, espresso, and green tea. If your preference is for dark or white tea, don't hesitate to appreciate it. The equivalent applies to home areas. The best news is that you canenjoy the infrequent glass of red wine during Phase 2. Red wine is a Sirtfood because of its substance of sirtuin-enacting polyphenols, particularly resveratrol and piceatannol, settling on it by a wide margin the best decision of mixed drink. However, with liquor itself effectively affecting our fat cells, control is still best, and all through Phase 2, we prescribe restricting your admission to one glass of red wine with a meal on a few days for every week.

Coming back To Three Meals

During Phase 1, you devoured only a couple of meals a day, which gave you bunches of adaptability over when you ate your meals. As we currently come back to a more standard al routine and the time-demonstrated example of three meals every day, it's a decent time to discuss breakfast.

Eating a decent breakfast sets us up for the afternoon, expanding our vitality and fixation levels. In term s of our digestion, eating prior keeps our glucose and fat levels under wraps. That breakfast is something to be thankful for is borne out by various examinations that ordinarily show that individuals who routinely eat breakfast are more reluctant to be overweight.

The explanation behind this is because of our interior body timekeepers. Our bodies anticipate that we should eat from the get-go fully expecting when we will be generally dynamic and satisfying fuel. However, on some random day, upwards of 33% of us will skip breakfast. It's a great side effect of our bustling present-day lives, and the recognition is that there isn't sufficient opportunity to eat well. However, as you will see, with the clever breakfasts we have spread out for you here, nothing could be further from reality. Regardless of whether it's the Sirtfood smoothie that can be flushed in a hurry, the premade Sirt muesli or the snappy and simple Sirtfood scram drained eggs/tofu, finding that an additional couple of moments toward the beginning of the day will harvest profits for your day as well as for your more extended term weight and wellbeing.

With Sirtfoods attempting to supercharge our vitality levels, there is much more to be picked up from getting an early morning hit of them to begin your day. This is accomplished by eating a Sirtfood-rich breakfast. Yet, particularly through the consideration of the green juice, which we suggest, you have either before anything else—in any event, thirty minutes before breakfast — or midmorning. From our clinical experience, we do get many reports of individuals who drink their gr squeeze first thing and don't feel hungry for several hours a while later. If this is the impact it has on you, it is impeccably ne to hold up a few hours before eating. Simply don't skip it.

On the other hand, you can commence your day with a decent breakfast; at that point, hold up a few hours before having the green juice. Be adaptable, and simply go with whatever works for you.

Sirtfood Bites

Concerning nibbling, you can accept the only choice available. There has been such a great amount of discussion about in the case of eating successive, littler meals are best for weight loss, or whether you should simply adhere to three adjusted meals a day. Truly, it doesn't generally make a difference.

How we have built the upkeep menu for you guarantees you will eat three even Sirtfood-rich meals every day, and you may discover you truly needn't bother with a tidbit. In any case, maybe you've been occupied in the workplace, working out, or running around with the children, and need something to hold you over to the following meal. Also, if that "small something" is going to give you a w ham m y of Sirtfood supplements and taste delightful, at that point, it's glad days. This is the reason we created our "Sirtfood chomps." These sharp little tidbits are a truly righteous treat made totally from Sirtfoods: dates, pecans, cocoa, additional virgin olive oil, and turmeric. For the days you need them, we suggest eating one, or a limit of two, every day.

"Sirtifying" Your Meals

We've seen that the main maintainable diets are ones of incorporation, not rejection. In any case, genuine progress goes past this—the diet must be good with cutting edge living. Regardless of whether it be the accommodation to satisfy the needs of our rushed lives or fitting in with our job as the bon vivant at dinner parties, the way we eat ought to be sans bother. You ought to have the option to make the most of your brilliant shine, rather than stressing over silly food requests and limitations.

What's so awesome about Sirtfoods is that they are extremely available, natural, and simple to remember for your diet. Here, as you overcome any issues between Phase 1 and routine eating, you will manufacture establishments for another, improved way of eating.

The key guideline is the thing that we call "Sirtifying" your meals. This is the place we take natural dishes, including numerous exemplary top picks. With some sharp trades and straightforward Sirtfood incorporations, we keep all the great taste, however, include a ton more goodness. All through Phase 2, you will see exactly how effectively this is accomplished.

Models incorporate our heavenly Sirtfood smoothie for the ideal in a hurried breakfast in a period starved world, and the straightforward change from wheat to buckwheat for adding additional taste and speed to the much-adored com stronghold food that is pasta. In the meantime, notable, adored dishes, for example, stew con carne and curry don't even n much change, with the customary recipes offering Sirtfood bonanzas. Also, who said cheap food implied terrible food? We consolidate the bona fide energetic kinds of a pizza and evacuate the blame when you make it yourself. There's no n to express goodbye to guilty pleasure either, as demonstrated by our flapjacks covered with berries and dim chocolate sauce. It's not even sweet, it's breakfast, and it's great for you. Straightforward changes: you keep on eating the foods you love while driving a healthy weight and prosperity. Furthermore, that is the dietary insurgency that is Sirtfoods.

Cooking for More

To grasp this, we are presently entering a "Sirtfoods for all" stage, where recipes start to take into account a greater number of mouths than one. Regardless of whether it be for family or companions, the new dinner recipes, just as the Sirtfood-stuffed soup we present in this phase are planned in light of cooking for four. What's more, for those as yet cooking for a couple of, why not exploit preparing group meals for fricasseeing to have meals prepared for one week from now?

What Can't You Eat?

Maintain a strategic distance from the accompanying foods while on the Sirtfood diet:

•	Processed foods – Salami, frankfurter, solidified foods, prepared to-eat foods, and stuffed organic product juices.

•	Sugary foods – Candies, cakes, pop, bundled organic product juice, doughnuts, baked goods, marshmallows, espresso or tea with cream and sugar, refined sugar, and so forth.

•	Fats and Oils – Butter, grease, and vegetable oil.

•	Starch – White rice and potato.

•	Trans Fats – Fries, burger, pizza, seared chicken, chips,

and rolls.

The Sirtfood diet is a genuinely basic diet to follow. It is separated into two phases, and each phase goes on for a week. Here's an example diet outline for Phase 1 that you can repeat for Phase 2 also. Investigate.

A 7-Day Sirtfood Diet Plan – Phase 1 and Phase 2

Phase 1: Week 1

Phase 1 of the Sirtfood diet proceeds in two phases – Stage 1 and Stage 2, each is going on for 3 and 4 days, separately. This is what to eat in the principal phase of Phase 1.

Stage 1 (Day 1 – Day 3) - *(1000 calories for every day)*

- 3 green juices every day

- 1 principle meal every day

- ½ or ¾ ounce of 85% dull chocolate

Principle Meal Options

- Red edamame, tomato, arugula, and buckwheat plate of mixed greens with olive oil dressing

- Celery, kale, and tricks plate of mixed greens with pecans and olive oil

Chicken bosom with arugula, kale, and pecans with strawberry and olive oil dressing

Stage 2 (Day 4 – Day 7) - *(1500 calories for every day)*

- 2 green juices every day
- 2 fundamental meals every day

Fundamental Meal Options

- Chicken stew
- Sirt museli
- Buckwheat noodles with soy lumps
- Strawberry, arugula, and pecan serving of mixed greens
- Grilled fish with red wine
- Waldorf serving of mixed greens

Phase 2: Week 2

During the subsequent week, you should repeat what you did in the principal week and keep up the weight loss.

After Phase 2

In the wake of finishing 14 days of the Sirtfood diet, this is what your diet plan should resemble:

- 3 adjusted Sirtfood-rich meals every day
- 1 Sirtfood green juice every day
- 1 or two Sirtfood snacks for each day

Are Sirtfoods The New Superfoods?

Indeed, Sirtfoods are the new superfoods. These actuate the fat-consuming gathering of qualities, SIRT1, and help improve wellbeing. These are mostly contained plant-based foods. They contain incredible phytonutrients that support digestion, forestall muscle loss, and converse numerous obesity-related medical problems.

Is the Sirtfood Diet Good for You?

Truly, the Sirtfood diet is beneficial for you. Research shows that foods remembered for this diet, similar to green tea, turmeric, and dim chocolate, have calming and cancer prevention agent properties. These foods help battle weight, coronary illness, hypertension, and stroke.

Studies led on lab creatures indicated that sirtuin-initiating foods increment life span, improve insulin affectability, consume increasingly fat, and lower the danger of malignant growth. Such encouraging outcomes on lab creatures and cell lines may not generally imply that the foods can likewise function admirably in people. However, the Sirtfood diet is an even diet plan that has great potential in supporting quick weight loss in people.

To guarantee safety, you should converse with your primary care physician or an enrolled dietitian before you start this diet. Your age, sex, BMI, clinical history, current prescription, and way of life will enable an authorized proficient at comprehending whether the Sirtfood diet will suit you. Keep in mind, and a diet plan may not generally suit all.

If you are new to drinking green juice, you may feel sick. Having just a couple of strong meals every day with 1000-1500 calories may likewise make you fractious, hungry, and irritable. Even though the diet has its advantages, it isn't intended for everybody.

Who Shouldn't Try the Sirtfood Diet?

Try not to attempt the Sirtfood diet if:

- Your specialist/nutritionist doesn't give you a green sign.
- You have hypoglycemia.
- You have a BMI under 30.
- You are on antidepressants.

- You are on different prescriptions.
- You have a convoluted clinical history.
- You experience the ill effects of IBD/IBS.
- If you are adversely affected by most foods referenced

in the Sirtfood's rundown.

Who Follows the Sirtfood Diet Already?

"Gossip has it" that Adele shed pounds by following the Sirtfood diet. Some different famous people into have attempted the diet are Jodie Kidd, Lorraine Pascale, and Sir Ben Ainslie. However, we don't have an immediate statement from these celebs or their delegates.

Sirtfood Recipes

1. Sirtfood Green Juice with Green Apple and Kiwi

Ingredients

- 1 green apple, hacked

- 2 kiwis, hacked

- 1 celery stem, hacked

- ½ a lime

- ½ tablespoon natural nectar

- A touch of pink Himalayan salt

- ½ teaspoon turmeric

The most effective method to prepare

1. Toss all the ingredients into a blender.

2. Blend well and pour it in a glass.

3. Drink up!

2. Sirtfood muesli In a Glass

Ingredients

- 1 cup muesli

- 1 cup milk or soy milk

- 1 cup yogurt or almond yogurt

- 10 huge strawberries

- A bunch of almonds

- ½ teaspoon vanilla concentrate

The most effective method to prepare

1. Toss portion of the strawberries and milk into a

blender.

2.   Blend well.

3.   Pour it into two tumblers.

4.   Add the muesli.

5.   Let it drench for 10 minutes.

6.   Top it with split strawberries and squashed almonds.

7.   Use a spoon to savor the delightful strawberry muesli.

Significant Questions Addressed Often

Are Sirtfoods Suitable for Children?

The Sirtfood diet is an amazing weight-loss diet and not intended for kids. Anyway, that doesn't imply that youngsters should pass up incorporating more Sirtfoods in their general diet for their surprising medical advantages and help them in accepting a reasonable and nutritious diet. A large number of the recipes have been created with families in mind, including kids' taste buds.

While most of Sirtfoods are amazingly healthy for youngsters, the green juice isn't suggested as it is extremely packed in fat-consuming Sirtfoods. The caffeine, as found in espresso and green tea, ought to be made preparations for as too with chilies. You may select to keep things milder for youngsters.

Would it be advisable for me to Exercise during Phase 1?

Doing some direct and ordinary exercise will upgrade the weight loss and medical advantages of Phase 1 of the diet. It is suggested you proceed with your ordinary degree of activity and physical movement through the initial seven days however remain inside your typical safe place as extremely drawn-out or too serious exercise may essentially put an excessive amount of weight on the body for this period. Tune in to your body and let the Sirtfoods accomplish the difficult work.

I'm Already Slim, Can I Still Follow the Diet?

Phase 1 of the Sirtfood Diet isn't suggested for any individual who is underweight. The ideal approach to see whether you are underweight is to compute your Body Mass Index or BMI. There are various BMI, for example, this one on the web. If your BMI is 17.5 or lower, Phase 1 of the diet isn't suggested. While numerous individuals want to be super-thin, actually being underweight can negatively affect numerous parts of your wellbeing, for example, a brought invulnerable system, a raised danger of debilitating of the bones (osteoporosis) and richness issues. All things considered, if you are underweight, it is suggested that you incorporate a lot of Sirtfoods into your diet to receive all their wellbeing rewards.

In any case, if you are thin with a BMI in the healthy scope of 20 to 25 by all methods, begin. You can, at present, get more fit, become progressively conditioned, and get enhancements in your vitality levels, appearance, and essentialness. The Sirtfood Diet is tied in with advancing wellbeing as much for what it's worth about getting more fit.

CHAPTER EIGHT

AFTER THE DIET

Getting more fit is sometimes very strenuous. However, dieters are likewise confronted with the way that situation is anything but favorable for them for long haul achievement. Analysts gauge that just around 20 percent of dieters keep up weight loss after a diet. Is it accurate to say that you will be one of them?

Step by Step Instructions to Maintain Weight Loss After a Diet

To build your odds of weight support after a diet, plan for a transitional phase after you arrive at your objective weight.

During this time, make moderate changes following your way of life and watch the consequences for the scale. Unexpected changes are probably going to cause weight recovery.

This transitional phase is additionally a decent time to recognize the eating propensities and exercise designs that you learned while dieting so you can keep up as long as possible. If you transform healthy diet propensities into a healthy way of life propensities, you're probably going to forestall weight recapture.

Specialists have discovered that dieters who keep the weight off for good are the individuals who keep on keeping up a low-fat diet with a lot of foods from the ground.

Ten Habits to Help You Maintain Your Weight

The ten propensities beneath will assist you with moving from the dieting phase through the transitional phase, lastly into the support phase, where your weight stays stable. To improve your odds of perpetual weight-loss achievement, attempt to fuse these ten propensities into your way of life as you travel through all phases of the dieting venture.

1.   Moderate weight loss works best. Doctors suggest that dieters lose close to one to two pounds every week. This moderate methodology assists patients with maintaining a strategic distance from wellbeing dangers related to extraordinary weight loss. It likewise permits the dieter to learn new eating propensities that will ensure their weight loss over the long haul. Segment control, healthy eating, ordinary exercise, and perusing dietary names are key aptitudes that you'll ace if you pick the more slow way to deal with weight loss.

2.   Make moderate progress out of the dieting stage. When you arrive at your objective weight, the most exceedingly terrible thing you can do is to continue your old eating propensities. Recollect that those are the eating propensities that caused the weight gain in any case. It is sensible to step by step increment caloric admission, yet specialists, for the most part, propose including just 200 calories for each week until your weight balances out.

3.   Stay associated with your wellsprings of help. Similar individuals who bolstered you in the dieting procedure will assist you with keeping up your weight loss. They are in the best situation to regard the size of your achievement and give you a delicate update if you forget about your prosperity. Speak with them and give them consent to offer an aware direction if necessary.

4.   Continue to challenge yourself with new objectives. Since you've aced probably the hardest test you'll ever confront, remain on your toes by defining another objective. It doesn't need to be identified with weight loss. Accomplishing both present moment and long haul objectives will assist you with keeping your certainty level high.

5.   Remain taught. Take healthy-cooking classes, go to wellbeing workshops, and take an interest in wellness fairs. Encircle yourself with tokens of what carrying on with a healthy life truly implies. You may likewise need to remain included on the web.

6.   Become a coach. Probably an ideal approach to remain instructed is to show your weight-loss aptitudes to an amateur. By turning into a coach, you'll be required to keep

steady over new research and patterns.

7.   Exercise. An investigation into changeless weight loss uncovers that activity is probably the best indicator of long haul achievement. Thirty to an hour of moderate exercise each day will keep both your body and psyche healthy.

8.   Eat breakfast. Studies have additionally discovered that individuals who eat breakfast are progressively effective at keeping the pounds under control. Ensure that your breakfast incorporates entire grains and a lean wellspring of protein.

9.   Weigh yourself. Keep a scale in your washroom and use it once per week. Studies show that checking your weight all the time is a training shared by individuals who effectively keep their weight off.

10.   Keep standard meetings with your social insurance group. Your human services supplier or enlisted dietician will have the option to quantify your muscle to fat ratio or assess your BMI to ensure that your numbers remain healthy. They will have the option to address medical problems that emerge when your body shape changes.

CHAPTER NINE

RECIPES

Sirtfood Juice

Ingredients:

- 2 enormous bunches (75g) kale

- An enormous bunch (30g) rocket

- A little bunch (5g) level leaf parsley

- A little bunch (5g) lovage leaves (discretionary)

- 2–3 enormous stems (150g) green celery, including its

leaves

- 1 small green apple

- Juice of 1 lemon

- 1 level tsp matcha green tea

Instructions:

- Mix the greens (kale, rocket, parsley, and lovage, if utilizing), at that point, juice them. We discover juicers can truly contrast in their proficiency at squeezing verdant vegetables, and you may need to re-squeeze the remainders before proceeding onward to different ingredients. The objective is to wind up with about 50ml of juice from the greens.

- Now juice the celery and apple. You can strip the lemon and put it through the juicer too, yet we think that it's a lot simpler just to crush the lemon by hand into the juice. By this stage, you ought to have around 250ml of juice altogether, maybe marginally more. It is just when the juice is made and prepared to serve that you include the matcha green tea.

- Pour a limited quantity of the juice into a glass. At that point, include the matcha and mix with a fork or teaspoon. We just use matcha in the initial two beverages of the day as it contains moderate measures of caffeine (a similar substance as a typical cup of tea). For individuals not accustomed to it, it might keep them alert whenever it's alcoholic. Once the matcha is broken, including the rest of the juice.

• Give it a last mix; at that point, your juice is prepared to drink. Don't hesitate to top up with plain water, as indicated by taste.

Sirt Muesli

If you need to make this in mass or set it up the prior night, combine the dry ingredients and store it in a sealed shut compartment. All you have to do the following day is include the strawberries and yogurt, and its all set.

Ingredients:

• 20g buckwheat pieces

• 10g buckwheat puffs

• 15g coconut pieces or dried up coconut

• 40g Medjool dates, hollowed and cleaved

• 15g pecans, cleaved

• 10g cocoa nibs

• 100g strawberries, hulled and cleaved

• 100g plain Greek yogurt (or veggie lover elective, for

example, soya or coconut yogurt)

Instructions:

Blend the entirety of the above ingredients (forget about the strawberries and yogurt if not serving straight away).

Fragrant Chicken Bosom With Kale, Red Onions, Tomato and Stew Salsa

Ingredients:

- 120g skinless, boneless chicken bosom
- 2 tsp ground turmeric
- Juice of ¼ lemon
- 1 tbsp additional virgin olive oil
- 50g kale, hacked
- 20g red onion, cut
- 1 tsp hacked new ginger
- 50g buckwheat
- For the salsa
- 130g tomato (around 1)

- 1 10,000 foot stew, finely slashed

- 1 tbsp tricks, finely hacked

- 5g parsley, finely hacked

- Juice of ¼ lemon

Instructions:

- To make the salsa, expel the eye from the tomato and hack it finely, taking consideration to keep however much of the fluid as could reasonably be expected. Blend in with the bean stew, tricks, parsley, and lemon juice. You could place everything in a blender, yet the final product is somewhat extraordinary.

- Heat the stove to 220ºC/gas 7. Marinate the chicken bosom in 1 teaspoon of the turmeric, the lemon juice, and a little oil. Leave for 5–10 minutes. Heat an ovenproof skillet until hot, at that point include the marinated chicken and cook for a moment or so on each side, until pale brilliant, at that point move to the broiler (place on a preparing plate if your container isn't ovenproof) for 8–10 minutes or until cooked through. Expel from the stove, spread with foil and leave to rest for 5 minutes before serving.

• Meanwhile, cook the kale in a liner for about 5 minutes. Fry the ginger and the red onions in a little oil; at that point, include the cooked kale and fry for one more moment. Cook the buckwheat as indicated by the parcel instructions with the rest of the teaspoon of turmeric. Serve nearby the chicken, vegetables, and salsa.

Sirtfood Nibbles

Ingredients:

• 120g pecans

• 30g dim chocolate (85 percent cocoa solids), broken into pieces; or cocoa nibs

• 250g Medjool dates pitted

• 1 tbsp. cocoa powder

• 1 tbsp. ground turmeric

• 1 tbsp. additional virgin olive oil

• The scratched seeds of 1 vanilla case or 1 tsp vanilla concentrate

• 1–2 tbsp. water

Instructions:

•   Place the pecans and chocolate in a food processor and procedure until you have a fine powder.

Include the various ingredients aside from the water and mix until the blend shapes a ball. You could conceivably need to include the water depending on the consistency of the blend – you don't need it to be excessively clingy.

•   Using your hands, structure the blend into reduced balls and refrigerate in an impermeable compartment for at any rate 1 hour before eating them. You could move a portion of the balls in some more cocoa or dried up a coconut to accomplish an alternate completion if you like. They will keep for as long as one week in your ice chest.

Asian Ruler Prawn Pan Sear With Buckwheat Noodles

Ingredients:

- 150g shelled crude ruler prawns, deveined

- 2 tsp. tamari (you can utilize soy sauce if you are not staying away from gluten)

- 2 tsp. additional virgin olive oil

- 75g soba (buckwheat noodles)

- 1 garlic clove, finely cleaved

- 1 elevated bean stew, finely cleaved

- 1 tsp. finely cleaved new ginger

- 20g red onions, cut

- 40g celery, cut and cut

- 75g green beans, cleaved

- 50g kale, generally cleaved

- 100ml chicken stock

- 5g lovage or celery leaves

Instructions:

- Heat a skillet over high heat; at that point, cook the

prawns in 1 teaspoon of the tamari and one teaspoon of the oil for 2–3 minutes. Move the prawns to a plate. Wipe the work out with kitchen paper, as you're going to utilize it once more.

• Cook the noodles in bubbling water for 5–8 minutes or as coordinated on the parcel. Channel and put in a safe spot.

• Meanwhile, fry the garlic, stew and ginger, red onion, celery, beans, and kale in the rest of the oil over medium-high heat for 2–3 minutes. Add the stock and bring to the bubble, at that point stew for a moment or two, until the vegetables are cooked yet at the same time crunchy.

• Add the noodles, prawns, and lovage/celery leaves to the dish, and take back to the bubble at that point expel from the heat and serve.

Strawberry Buckwheat Tabouleh

Ingredients:

• 50g buckwheat

• 1 tbsp. ground turmeric

• 80g avocado

• 65g tomato

- 20g red onion

- 25g Medjool dates pitted

- 1 tbsp. escapades

- 30g parsley

- 100g strawberries, hulled

- 1 tbsp additional virgin olive oil

- Juice of ½ lemon

- 30g rocket

Instructions:

- Cook the buckwheat with the turmeric, as indicated by the parcel instructions. Channel and keep to the other side to cool.

- Finely slash the avocado, tomato, red onion, dates, tricks, and parsley and blend in with the cool buckwheat. Cut the strawberries and delicately blend into the serving of mixed greens with the oil and lemon juice. Serve on a bed of rocket.

Marinated Baked Cod With Stir-Fried Greens

Ingredients:

- 3 1/2 teaspoons (20g) miso
- 1 tablespoon mirin
- 1 tablespoon extra-virgin olive oil
- 1 x 7-ounce (200g) skinless cod filet
- 1/8 cup (20g) red onion, cut
- 3/8 cup (40g) celery, cut
- 2 garlic cloves, finely cleaved
- 1 Thai bean stew, finely slashed
- 1 teaspoon finely cleaved new ginger
- 3/8 cup (60g) green beans
- 3/4 cup (50g) kale, generally cleaved
- 1 teaspoon sesame seeds
- 2 tablespoons (5g) parsley, generally cleaved
- 1 tablespoon of tamari
- 1/4 cup (40g) buckwheat
- 1 teaspoon ground turmeric

Instructions:

Blend the miso, mirin, and one teaspoon of the oil. Rub everywhere throughout the cod and leave to marinate for 30 minutes. Heat the broiler to 425oF (220oC).

Prepare the cod for 10 minutes.

In the interim, heat a larger skillet or wok with the rest of the oil. Include the onion and pan-fried food for a couple of moments; at that point, include the celery, garlic, stew, ginger, green beans, and kale. Hurl and fry until the kale is cooked. Add a little water to the dish to help the cooking procedure.

Cook the buckwheat as indicated by the bundle instructions along with the turmeric.

Include the sesame seeds, parsley, and tamari to the sautéed food and present with the buckwheat and fish.

Sirtfood Bites

Ingredients:

- 1 cup (120g) pecans

- 1 ounce (30g) dull chocolate (85 percent cocoa solids), broken into pieces; or 1/4 cup cocoa nibs

- 9 ounces (250g) Medjool dates, pitted

- 1 tablespoon cocoa powder

- 1 tablespoon ground turmeric

- 1 tablespoon additional virgin olive oil

- The scratched seeds of 1 vanilla unit or one teaspoon vanilla concentrate

- 1 to 2 tablespoons water

Instructions:

Spot the pecans and chocolate in a food processor and procedure until you have a fine powder.

Include the various ingredients aside from the water and mix until the blend frames a ball. You might need to include the water depending on the consistency of the blend—you don't need it to be excessively clingy.

Utilizing your hands, structure the blend into reduced balls and refrigerate in a water/air proof compartment for in any event 1 hour before eating them.

You could move a portion of the balls in some more cocoa or dried coconut to accomplish an alternate completion if you like. They will keep for as long as one week in your refrigerator.

Sirt Super Salad

Ingredients:
- 1 3⁄4 ounces (50g) arugula
- 1 3⁄4 ounces (50g) endive leaves
- 3 1⁄2 ounces (100g) smoked salmon cuts
- 1⁄2 cup (80g) avocado, stripped, stoned, and cut
- 1⁄2 cup (50g) celery including leaves, cut
- 1⁄8 cup (20g) red onion, cut

- 1/8 cups (15g) pecans, cleaved

- 1 tablespoon escapades

- 1 enormous Medjool date, hollowed and slashed

- 1 tablespoon additional virgin olive oil

- Juice of 1/4 lemon

- 1/4 cup (10g) parsley, hacked

Instructions:

Spot the serving of mixed greens, leaves on a plate, or in a huge bowl.

Combine all the rest of the ingredients and serve on the leaves.

Sweet-smelling Chicken Breast with Kale and Red Onions and a Tomato and Chili Salsa

Ingredients:

- 1/4 pound (120g) skinless, boneless chicken bosom

- 2 teaspoons ground turmeric

- Juice of 1/4 lemon

- 1 tablespoon additional virgin olive oil

- 3⁄4 cup (50g) kale, slashed

- 1⁄8 cup (20g) red onion, cut

- 1 teaspoon slashed new ginger

- 1⁄3 cup (50g) buckwheat

For the Salsa

- 1 medium tomato (130g)

- 1 Thai bean stew, finely hacked

- 1 tablespoon escapades, finely hacked

- 2 tablespoons (5g) parsley, finely slashed

- Juice of 1⁄4 lemon

Instructions:

To make the salsa, expel the eye from the tomato and hack it finely, taking consideration to keep however much of the fluid as could reasonably be expected. Blend in with the stew, escapades, parsley, and lemon juice. You could place everything in a blender. However, the final product is somewhat extraordinary.

Heat the stove to 425ºF (220ºC). Marinate the chicken bosom in 1 teaspoon of the turmeric, the lemon juice, and a little oil. Leave for 5 to 10 minutes.

Heat an ovenproof skillet until hot, at that point include the marinated chicken and cook for a moment or so on each side, until pale brilliant, at that point move to the broiler (place on a preparing plate if your skillet isn't ovenproof) for 8 to 10 minutes or until cooked through. Expel from the stove, spread with foil, and leave to rest for 5 minutes before serving.

Then, cook the kale in a liner for about 5 minutes. And ensure to fry the ginger and red onions in a little oil as desired, at that point include the cooked kale and fry for one more moment.

Cook the buckwheat as indicated by the bundle instructions with the rest of the teaspoon of turmeric. Serve close by the chicken, vegetables, and salsa.

Asian Shrimp Stir-Fry With Buckwheat Noodles

Ingredients:

- 1/3 pound (150g) shelled gigantic crude shrimp, deveined

- 2 teaspoons tamari (you can utilize soy sauce if you are not maintaining a strategic distance from gluten)

- 2 teaspoons additional virgin olive oil

- 3 ounces (75g) soba (buckwheat noodles)

- 2 garlic cloves, finely cleaved

- 1 Thai bean stew, finely slashed

- 1 teaspoon finely cleaved new ginger

- 1/8 cup (20g) red onions, cut

- 1/2 cup (45g) celery including leaves, cut and cut, with leaves put in a safe spot

- 1/2 cup (75g) green beans, cleaved

- 3/4 cup (50g) kale, generally hacked

- 1/2 cup (100ml) chicken stock

Instructions:

Heat a skillet over high heat; at that point, cook the shrimp in 1 teaspoon of the tamari and one teaspoon of the oil for 2 to 3 minutes.

Move the shrimp to a plate. Wipe the work out with a paper towel, as you're going to utilize it once more.

Cook the noodles in bubbling water for 5 to 8 minutes or as coordinated on the bundle. Channel and put in a safe spot.

In the meantime, fry the garlic, stew, ginger, red onion, celery (yet not the leaves), green beans, and kale in the remaining tamari and oil over medium-high heat for 2 to 3 minutes. Add the stock and heat to the point of boiling, at that point stew for a moment or two, until the vegetables are cooked yet at the same time crunchy.

Include the shrimp, noodles, and celery leaves to the skillet, heat back to the point of boiling, at that point expel from the heat and serve.

Strawberry Buckwheat Tabbouleh

Ingredients:

- 1/3 cup (50g) buckwheat
- 1 tablespoon ground turmeric
- 1/2 cup (80g) avocado
- 3/8 cup (65g) tomato
- 1/8 cup (20g) red onion
- 1/8 cup (25g) Medjool dates, pitted
- 1 tablespoon tricks
- 3/4 cup (30g) parsley
- 2/3 cup (100g) strawberries, hulled
- 1 tablespoon extra-virgin olive oil
- Juice of 1/2 lemon
- 1 ounce (30g) arugula

Instructions:

Cook the buckwheat with the turmeric as per the bundle instructions.

Channel and put aside to cool.

Finely hack the avocado, tomato, red onion, dates, tricks, and parsley and blend in with the cool buckwheat.

Cut the strawberries and tenderly blend in to the plate of mixed greens with the oil and lemon juice. Serve on a bed of arugula.

Sirtfood Green Juice

Ingredients:

- 2 enormous bunches (around 2 1/2 ounces or 75g) kale

- An enormous bunch (1 ounce or 30g) arugula

- An extremely little bunch (about 1/4 ounce or 5g) level leaf parsley

- 2 to 3 enormous celery stems (5 1/2 ounces or 150g), including leaves

- 1/2 medium green apple

- 1/2-to 1-inch (1 to 2.5 cm) bit of new ginger

- Juice of 1/2 lemon

- 1/2 level teaspoon matcha powder

Instructions:

Blend the greens (kale, arugula, and parsley). At that point, juice them. We find that juicers can truly contrast in their proficiency at squeezing verdant vegetables, and you may need to juice the leftovers before proceeding onward to different ingredients. The objective is to wind up with around two liquid ounces or near 1/4 cup (50ml) of juice from the greens.

Squeeze the celery, apple, and ginger.

You can strip the lemon and put it through the juicer also, however, we think that it's a lot simpler just to crush the lemon by hand into the juice. By this stage, you ought to have around 1 cup (250ml) of juice altogether, maybe somewhat more.

It is just when the juice is made and prepared to serve that you include the matcha. Pour a modest quantity of the juice into a glass; at that point, include the matcha and mix overwhelmingly with a fork or teaspoon.

Once the match is broken down, including the rest of the juice, give it a last mix; at that point, your juice is prepared to drink. Don't hesitate to top up with plain water, as per taste.

Mixed Omelet Toast Topper

Ingredients

- 2 eggs

- 1 tsp. crème fraîche

- 25g cheddar, ground

- Small pack chive, clipped

- 1 spring onion, cut

- 1 tsp. oil

- 3-4 cherry tomatoes, split

- 2 cuts dried up bread, toasted

Instructions:

Beat eggs, crème fraîche, cheddar, and chives together with a touch of flavoring. Heat oil in a skillet, at that point, relax spring onion for a couple of mins. Include tomatoes and warm through, at that point pour in egg blend. Cook over low heat, mixing, until eggs are simply set. Heap over toast.

One-dish summer eggs

Ingredients

- 1 tsp. olive oil
- 400g courgettes (around two huge ones), slashed into little lumps
- 200g/7oz pack cherry tomatoes, split
- 1 garlic clove, squashed
- 2 eggs
- Few basil leaves, to serve

Instructions:

Heat the oil in a non-stick skillet, at that point, including the courgettes. Fry for 5 mins, mixing now and then until they begin to relax, including the tomatoes and garlic, at that point cook for a couple of mins more. Mix in a touch of flavoring; at that point, make two holes in the blend and split in the eggs.

Spread the skillet with a cover or a sheet of foil. At that point, cook for 2-3 mins until the eggs are done exactly as you would prefer. Dissipate over a couple of basil leaves and present with dried-up bread.

Veggie lover cook

Ingredients

- 1 big potato (unpeeled)
- 1 1/2 tablespoon nutty spread
- For the berries and mushrooms
- 14 cherry tomatoes
- Jojoba oil
- 2 tsp. pecan syrup
- 1 teaspoon soy sauce
- 1/4 tsp. smoked paprika
- 1 enormous Portobello mushroom, cut
- For Your mixed tofu
- 349g pack luxurious tofu
- 2 tablespoons nourishing enhancement
- 1/2 tsp. turmeric

- 1 tsp. garlic, squashed

- To work

- 4 veggie lover frankfurters (we used Dee's leek and pumpkin)

- 1 x 200g can heated beans

Instructions:

- Cook the curry whole in a major bowl of water, at that point stew for 10 mins at that point channel, and let it cool. Strip the skin off then coarsely grind. Blend utilizing all the nutty spread and season well. Put aside in the cooler until required.

- Heat stove to 200C/180C fan/gas 6. Set the cherry tomatoes on a preparing dish, sprinkle with 2 tsp. Sunflower oil, season, and heat for 30 mins or until the skins have irritated and start to roast. Cook the beans and stew following the directions on the bundle with the goal that they're set up to work incorrectly precisely the same time frame as the mixed tofu.

- Meanwhile, join the maple syrup, soy sauce, and 1/4 tsp smoked paprika together in a colossal bowl; at that point, include the hacked mushroom and hurl to cover from the blend. Leave to remain as you pour two tsp sunflower oil to some non-stick skillet and bring this up into medium heat. Fry the mushroom till simply starting to turn gold however not scorched. Bend onto a plate and keep warm before serving.

•	Place one tablespoon oil to the skillet and afterward include spoonfuls of the potato blend - you should have around

•	Fry for 3-4 mins each side at that point spurt on kitchen paper.

•	Crumble the tofu to your skillet and afterward dissipate on the rest of the ingredients alongside a phenomenal spot of pepper and salt. If the skillet appears to be somewhat dry, include a spot more oil. Fry until the tofu is separated into bits, pleasantly covered in the flavoring and warm through.

•	Split everything between two plates and present with a hot cup of tea created with soy milk.

Coconut and Banana Sandwiches

Ingredients

- 150g plain flour

- 2 tsp. coconut powder

- 3 tablespoons brilliant caster sugar

- 400ml may coconut milk, shaken well

- Vegetable oil, for broiling

- 1-2 bananas, daintily cut

- 2 energy natural products, substance scooped out

Instructions:

1. Filter the flour and preparing powder into a bowl and mix in 2 tablespoons of the sugar and a touch of salt. Empty the coconut milk into a bowl, at that point race to consolidate in any fat that is part, at that point, step out 300ml to a container. Mix the milk bit by bit into the flour blend to make a smooth player, at that point, or whizz everything in a blender.

2. Heating a shallow skillet or level frying pan and brush it with oil. Utilize two tbsp. Of hitter to create every flapjack, skillet at once - some more will make it precarious to flip them. Push 4-5 pieces of banana to every hotcake and cook until bubbles start to pop the surface, and the edges seem dry. They'll be more delicate than egg-based hotcakes, like this

turn them over cautiously and cook other regions for 1 minute. Copy to create 8-10 hotcakes.

3. Place the remaining coconut milk and sugar in a little container. Include a touch of salt and stew until the blend thickens to the consistency of single cream. Utilize this as a sauce for those wieners and spoon over a portion of the fire seeds.

Summer porridge

Ingredients

- 300ml almond milk
- 200g blueberries
- 1/2 tablespoon pecan syrup
- 2 tbsp. chia seeds
- 100g kind sized oats
- 1 kiwi berry, cut into pieces
- 50g pomegranate seeds
- 2 tsp blended seeds

Instructions:

1. In A blender, rush the milk, blueberries, and maple syrup before the milk turns purple. Spot the chia and oats at a blending bowl; at that point, fill the skillet and mix truly well. Leave to bubble for 5 mins, mixing every so often, until the fluid has expended, alongside the oats and chia expand and thicken.

2. Mix once more, at that point, split between 2 dishes. Organize the natural product on top, and afterward dissipate over the seeds that are blended. I will keep in the fridge for one day. Supplement the fixings only preceding serving.

Vegetarian Tomato and coriander hotcakes

Ingredients

- 140g white self-rising flour

- 1 teaspoon soya flour

- 400ml soya milk

- Vegetable oil, for the grill

For the garnish

- 2 tablespoons vegetable oil

- 250g button mushrooms

- 250g cherry tomatoes, divided

- 2 tablespoon soya cream or soya milk

- Sizable number pine nuts

- Snipped chives, to work

Instructions:

1. Filter the flours alongside a spot of salt into a blender. Include the soya milk and blend to create a smooth hitter.

2. Heating only a little oil in a moderate non-stick skillet till hot. Pour around three tablespoons of the player to the skillet and cook over moderate heat until bubbles show up on the outside of the flapjack. Flip the flapjack over with a palette blade and cook on the opposite side until brilliant earthy colored. Repeat with the rest of the player, keeping the cooked hotcakes warm as you move. You may make about 8.

3. The garnish, heat the oil in a skillet. Cook the mushrooms until delicate; at that point, include the tomatoes and cook for a couple of mins. Pour from the soya cream or milk and pine nuts, at that point cook till mixed. Split the sausage between two plates, at that point, spoon on the berries and mushrooms. Disperse with chives.

Vegetarian Granola

Ingredients

- 400g kind sized oats

- 2 tsp. cinnamon

- 150g dried apple, generally cut

- 150g coconut oil, liquefied

- 250g pack blended nuts, generally cleaved

- 100ml pecan syrup

Instructions:

1. Heating Oven to 180C/160C fan/gas 4. Line two huge heating plates with preparing material. Combine the entirety of the ingredients aside from the maple syrup. Spread the granola out onto the plate and sprinkle over the maple syrup.

2. Prepare from the grill for 20 mins, mixing the granola pleasantly partially through so it cooks equitably. Leave to cool before putting away in a Kilner container or impermeable holder.

Mexican Beans and Avocado Toast

Ingredients

- 270g cherry tomatoes, quartered

- 1 white or red onion, finely hacked

- 1/2 lime, squeezed

- 4 tablespoons olive oil

- 2 garlic cloves, squashed

- 1 teaspoon ground cumin

- 2 tsp. Chipotle glue or 1 tsp. stew drops

- 2 x 400g jars dark beans, depleted

- Little pack coriander, slashed

- 4 cuts bread

- 1 avocado, finely hacked

Instructions:

1. Blend the berries, 1/4 onion, lime juice, and one tablespoon oil and put in a safe spot. Fry the remainder of the onion in 2 tablespoons oil until it starts to mollify. Include the garlic, fry for one moment, at that point include the cumin and chipotle and sautéed food until sweet-smelling. Indication in the

vegetables and a scramble of water, cook and mix tenderly until heated through. Mix in most of the tomato blend and cook one moment, season well, and incorporate most of the coriander.

2. Toast the bread and topping with the staying one tablespoon oil. Set a piece on each plate and heap a couple of beans on top. Sort out certain bits of avocado on top, and afterward disperse the rest of the tomato blend and coriander leaves to work.

Three-Grain Porridge

This Nutritious breakfast, produced using toasted oatmeal, grain, and wheat, is excessively simple to create and might be kept up for as long as a half-year

Ingredients

- 300g oatmeal
- 300g chips drop
- 300g grain drops

- Agave nectar and slashed strawberries, to serve (discretionary)

Instructions:

1. Working In clusters, toast the oatmeal, chips, and grain at a major, dry skillet for 5 mins until brilliant, at that point leave to cool and store in an impermeable holder.

2. At the point when you might want to expend that, simply mix 50g of this porridge blend in a pot with 300ml water or milk. Cook for 5 mins, blending incidentally, at that point top with a spoonful of nectar and tomatoes, if you like (discretionary). It will save for six weeks.

Daylight Smoothie

Ingredients

- 50zml lettuce juice, chilled
- 200g pineapple (canned or new)
- Two bananas, broken into lumps
- Little piece ginger, stripped

- 20g cashew nuts juice lime

Instructions:

1. Spot the ingredients at a blender and whizz until smooth. Drink legitimately away or fill a container to drink progressing. Will keep in the fridge for a solitary day.

Veggie Lover Smoothie

Ingredients

- 100ml (1/4 tall glass) cherry Juice

- 200ml (1/2 tall glass) unsweetened soya milk

- 1 cherry soya yogurt

- 3 tablespoons or 50g firm smooth tofu

- 75g (1 empty yogurt pot) solidified cherry

- 2 tbsp. porridge oat

Instructions:

1. Evaluate every one of the segments just or use a tall glass alongside your unfilled yogurt pot for rate - they don't should be exact. Spot them in a blender and rush until smooth. Pour one tall glass (you will have enough to get a high up) or two

short tumblers.

Kiwi Organic Product Smoothie

Ingredients

- 3 stripped kiwi berry

- 1 mango, stripped, stoned and cut

- 500ml lemon juice

- 1 banana, cut

Instructions:

Place all the ingredients at a blender and crush until they are smooth at that point fill two tall glasses.

The Sirtfood Diet Salmon Super-Serving of Mixed Greens

Ingredients

- 50 g rocket

- 50 g chicory leaves

- 100 g smoked salmon cuts

- 80 g avocado, stripped, stoned and cut

- 15 g pecans, slashed

- 1 tbsp. escapades

- 1 enormous Medjool date, hollowed and hacked

- 1 tbsp. additional virgin olive oil juice of 1/4 of a lemon

- 10 g parsley, hacked

- 10 g lovage or celery leaves, hacked

- 40 g celery, cut

- 20 g red onion, cut

Instructions:

- Place the serving of mixed greens leaves on a plate or in a huge bowl. Combine all the rest of the ingredients and serve on the leaves.

- For a lentil Sirt super plate of mixed greens, supplant the smoked salmon with 100g tinned green lentils or cooked Puy lentils.

- For a chicken Sirt super plate of mixed greens, supplant the smoked salmon with a cut cooked chicken bosom.

- For a fish Sirt super plate of mixed greens, supplant the

smoked salmon with tinned fish (purchased in saline solution or oil as per inclination).

The Sirtfood Diet Green Juice Salad

Ingredients

- Juice of ½ lemon
- 1 cm ginger ground
- Salt and pepper to taste
- 1 tablespoon olive oil
- 2 bunches kale cut
- 1 bunch rocket
- 1 tablespoon parsley
- 2 celery sticks cut
- ½ green apple cut
- 6 pecan parts

Instructions:

1. Put the lemon juice, ginger, salt, pepper, and olive oil in a jam container and shake to consolidate.

2. Place the kale in an enormous blow away and pour the

dressing. Back rub the dressing into the kale for one moment.

3.   Add the various ingredients and combine them all.

Chicken Curry

Ingredients

*   1 red onion generally slashed

*   3 garlic cloves generally slashed

*   2 cm new ginger stripped and generally slashed

*   2 teaspoons garam masala

*   2 teaspoons ground cumin

*   2 teaspoons ground turmeric

*   1 cinnamon stick discretionary

*   6 cardamom cases discretionary

*   1 tablespoon olive oil

*   8 boneless skinless chicken thighs (or six chicken chests), cut into bitesize lumps

*   1 x 400ml tin coconut milk

*   2 tablespoons new coriander slashed (in addition to extra for embellish)

*   200 g buckwheat earthy colored rice or basmati rice to

serve

Instructions

1.   Place the onion, garlic, and ginger in a food processor and barrage until it is glue. Then again, you can do this with a hand blender, or if you don't have one, simply cleave these three ingredients finely and proceed as underneath.

2.   Add the garam masala, cumin, and turmeric to the glue and mix. Put in a safe spot.

3.   Put one tablespoon of olive oil in a wide, profound dish (in a perfect world non-stick). Heat the dish on high heat for one moment and afterward include the cleaved up chicken thighs. Sautéed food the chicken on high heat for 2 minutes, at that point, turn the heat and include the curry glue. Permit the chicken to cook in the glue for 3 minutes and afterward include a large portion of the coconut milk (200ml), in addition to the cinnamon and cardamom (if utilizing). Bring to the come and afterward turn and permit to stew for 30 minutes until the curry sauce is thick and heavenly!

4.   If the curry begins to get dry, include a sprinkle more coconut milk. You may not require everything, except if you like a somewhat increasingly saucy curry, by all methods include the parcel!

5.   While the curry is cooking, make your backup (buckwheat/rice) and any side dishes.

6.   When the curry is prepared, include the hacked coriander and serve quickly with buckwheat or rice and a pleasant glass of chilled white wine.

Prepared Potatoes with Spicy Chickpea Stew

Ingredients

*   4-6 preparing potatoes pricked everywhere

*   2 tablespoons olive oil

*   2 red onions finely hacked

*   4 cloves garlic ground or squashed

*   2 cm ginger ground

- 1 to 2 teaspoons stew chips (relying upon how hot you like things)

- 2 tablespoons cumin seeds

- 2 tablespoons turmeric

- Splash of water

- 2 x 400g tins hacked tomatoes

- 2 x 400g kidney beans if you lean toward including the chickpea water.

- 2 yellow peppers or whatever shading you like!

- 2 tablespoons parsley in addition to extra for decorating

- Salt and pepper to taste discretionary

- Side serving of mixed greens discretionary

Instructions

1. Preheat the broiler to 200C; in the meantime, you can set up the entirety of your ingredients.

2. When the grill is hot enough, placed your heating potatoes in the stove and cook for 1 hour or until they are done how you like them. (Don't hesitate to utilize your

ordinary heated potato method if it's not quite the same as mine!)

3.   Once the potatoes are in the broiler, place the olive oil and cleaved red onion in a huge wide pan and cook tenderly, with the top on for 5 minutes, until the onions are delicate yet not earthy colored.

4.   Remove the top and include garlic, ginger, cumin, and bean stew. Cook for a further moment on low heat. At that point, include the turmeric and a little sprinkle of water and cook for one more moment, taking consideration not to let the container get excessively dry.

5.   Next, include the tomatoes, cocoa powder (or cacao), chickpeas (counting the chickpea water), and yellow pepper. Then stew on a low heat for about 40 minutes until the sauce is thick and greasy (however, don't allow it to consume!). The stew ought to be done at generally a similar time as the potatoes.

6.   Finally, mix in the two tablespoons of parsley, and some salt and pepper if you wish, and serve the stew on the heated potatoes, maybe with a straightforward side plate of mixed greens.

Kale and Red Onion Dhal with Buckwheat

Ingredients

- 1 tablespoon olive oil

- 1 little red onion cut

- 3 garlic cloves ground or squashed

- 2 cm ginger ground

- 1 winged creature eye bean stew deseeded and finely slashed (more if you like things hot!)

- 2 teaspoons turmeric

- 2 teaspoons of masala

- 500 ml of coconut milk

- 200 ml of water

- 100 g kale or spinach

- 160 g buckwheat or earthy colored rice

Instructions

1.   Put the olive oil in a huge, profound pot and include the cut onion. Cook on low heat, with the top on for 5 minutes until relaxed.

2.   Add the garlic, ginger, and stew and cook for one progressively minute.

3.   Add the turmeric, garam masala, and a sprinkle of water and cook for one progressively minute.

4.   Add the coconut milk, red lentils, and 220ml water (do this significantly filling the coconut milk can with water and tipping it into the pot).

5.   Mix everything completely and cook for 20 minutes over a tenderly heat with the top on. Mix sporadically and include somewhat more water if the dhal begins to stick.

6.   After 20 minutes, including the kale, mix completely

and supplant the cover, cook for a further 5 minutes (1-2 minutes if you use spinach!)

7.   About 15 minutes before the curry is prepared, place the buckwheat in a medium pan, and include a lot of bubbling water. Take the water back to the bubble and cook for 10 minutes (or somewhat more if you favor your buckwheat gentler. Channel the buckwheat in a strainer and present with the dhal.

Ruler Prawn Stir Fry with Buckwheat Noodles

Ingredients

- 300 g buckwheat/soba noodles attempt to get 100% buckwheat if you can
- 2 tablespoons additional virgin olive oil
- 1 red onion cut daintily
- 2 sticks of celery cut
- 100 g kale generally cleaved
- 100 g green beans cleaved
- 3 cm ginger ground

- 3 garlic cloves ground or finely cleaved

- 1 10,000 foot stew seeds/layers evacuated and hacked finely (or more to taste)

- 600 g lord prawns

- 2 tablespoons tamari/soy sauce in addition to extra for serving

- 2 tablespoons parsley cleaved

Instructions

1. Cook the noodles for about 5 minutes or till when they are done just as you would prefer—Channel, flush in cool water. Shower over a little olive oil, blend and put in a safe spot.

2. While the noodles are cooking, set up the remainder of the ingredients.

3. In a wok or enormous skillet, fry the red onion and celery in a little olive oil over a delicate heat for 3 minutes until delicate, at that point, include the kale and green beans and fry over medium-high heat for 3 minutes.

4.   Turn the heat again and include the ginger, garlic, bean stew, and prawns. Fry about 4 minutes until the prawns are hot completely through.

5.   Add the noodles, soy sauce (or tamari), and cook for one increasingly minute until the noodles are warm once more. Sprinkle with parsley and serve.

Turmeric Chicken and Kale Salad With Honey Lime Dressing

If getting ready early, dress the plate of mixed greens 10 minutes before serving. Chicken can be supplanted with meat mince, hacked prawns, or fish. Vegans could utilize cleaved mushrooms or cooked quinoa.

Ingredients

For the chicken

- 1 teaspoon of coconut oil

- ½ medium earthy colored onion, diced

- 250-300 g/9 oz. chicken mince or diced up chicken thighs
- 1 huge garlic clove, finely diced
- 1 teaspoon turmeric powder
- 1teaspoon lime get-up-and-go
- Juice of ½ lime
- ½ teaspoon salt + pepper

For the plate of mixed greens

- 8 broccolini stalks
- 2 tablespoons of pumpkin seeds
- 3 huge kale leaves, stems expelled and cleaved
- ½ avocado, cut
- Handful of new coriander leaves, hacked
- Handful of new parsley leaves, hacked

For the dressing

- 3 tablespoons lime juice
- 1 little garlic clove, finely diced or ground
- 3 tablespoons extra-virgin olive oil
- 1 teaspoon crude nectar
- ½ teaspoon wholegrain or Dijon mustard

- ½ teaspoon ocean salt and pepper

Instructions

1. Heat the coconut oil in a little skillet over medium-high heat. Include the onion and sauté medium heat for 4-5 minutes, until brilliant. Include the chicken mince and garlic and mix for 2-3 minutes over medium-high heat, breaking it separated.

2. Include the turmeric, lime pizzazz, lime squeeze, salt, and pepper and cook, blending as often as possible, for a further 3-4 minutes. Put the cooked mince in a safe spot.

3. While the chicken is cooking, carry a little pot of water to bubble. Include the broccolini and cook for 2 minutes. Wash under virus water and cut into 3-4 pieces each.

4. Add the pumpkin seeds to the skillet from the chicken and toast over medium heat for 2 minutes, mixing now and again to forestall consuming—season with somewhat salt. Put in a safe spot. Crude pumpkin seeds are additionally fine to

utilize.

5. Spot hacked kale in a plate of mixed greens astound and pour the dressing. Utilizing your hands, hurl, and back rub the kale with the dressing. This will relax the kale, sort of like what citrus juice does to fish or meat carpaccio – it 'cooks' it marginally.

6. At last, hurl through the cooked chicken, broccolini, new herbs, pumpkin seeds, and avocado cuts.

Buckwheat Noodles with Chicken Kale and Miso Dressing

Ingredients

For the noodles

- 2-3 bunches of kale leaves

- 150 g/5 oz of buckwheat noodles

- 3-4 shiitake mushrooms, cut

- 1 teaspoon coconut oil or ghee

- 1 earthy colored onion, finely diced

- 1 medium unfenced chicken bosom, cut or diced

- 1 long red bean stew, meagerly cut (seeds in or out contingent upon how hot you like it)

- 2 enormous garlic cloves, finely diced

- 2-3 tablespoons Tamari sauce (sans gluten soy sauce)

For the miso dressing

- 1½ tablespoon new natural miso

- 1 tablespoon Tamari sauce

- 1 tablespoon extra-virgin olive oil

- 1 tablespoon lemon or lime juice

- 1 teaspoon sesame oil (discretionary)

Instructions

1. Carry a medium pan of water to bubble. Include the kale and cook for one moment, until somewhat withered. Expel and put in a safe spot yet save the water and take it back to the bubble. Include the soba noodles and cook as indicated by the bundle instructions (for the most part, around 5 minutes). Wash under virus water and put it in a safe spot.

2. Meanwhile, sear the shiitake mushrooms in a little ghee or coconut oil (about a teaspoon) for 2-3 minutes, until delicately caramelized on each side. Sprinkle with ocean salt and put it in a safe spot.

3. In a similar skillet, heat more coconut oil or ghee over medium-high heat. Sauté onion and bean stew for 2-3 minutes and afterward include the chicken pieces. Cook 5 minutes over medium heat, mixing a few times, at that point include the garlic, tamari sauce, and a little sprinkle of water. Cook for a further 2-3 minutes, mixing now and again until chicken is cooked through.

4. At last, include the kale and soba noodles and hurl through the chicken to heat up.

5. Mix the miso dressing and sprinkle over the noodles directly toward the finish of cooking, along these lines you will keep every one of those gainful probiotics in the miso alive and dynamic.

Asian King Prawn Stir-Fry with Buckwheat Noodles

Ingredients:

- 150g shelled crude ruler prawns, deveined
- 2 tsp tamari (you can utilize soy sauce if you are not staying away from gluten)
- 2 tsp additional virgin olive oil
- 75g soba (buckwheat noodles)
- 1 garlic clove, finely slashed
- 1 elevated bean stew, finely cleaved
- 1 tsp finely slashed new ginger
- 20g red onions, cut
- 40g celery, cut and cut
- 75g green beans, slashed
- 50g kale, generally slashed
- 100ml chicken stock
- 5g lovage or celery leaves

Instructions:

Heat a skillet over high heat; at that point, cook the prawns in

1 teaspoon of the tamari and one teaspoon of the oil for 2–3 minutes. Move the prawns to a plate. Wipe the work out with kitchen paper, as you're going to utilize it once more.

Cook the noodles in bubbling water for 5–8 minutes or as coordinated on the parcel. Channel and put in a safe spot.

In the meantime, fry the garlic, stew and ginger, red onion, celery, beans, and kale in the rest of the oil over medium-high heat for 2–3 minutes. Add the stock and bring to the bubble, at that point stew for a moment or two, until the vegetables are cooked yet at the same time crunchy.

Include the prawns, noodles, and lovage/celery leaves to the skillet, take back to the bubble at that point expel from the heat and serve.

Heated Salmon Salad with Creamy Mint Dressing

Heating the salmon in the stove makes this plate of mixed

greens so basic.

Ingredients

- 1 salmon filet (130g)
- 40g blended plate of mixed greens leaves
- 40g youthful spinach leaves
- 2 radishes, cut and daintily cut
- 5cm piece (50g) cucumber, cut into lumps
- 2 spring onions, cut and cut
- 1 little bunch (10g) parsley, generally hacked

For the dressing:

- 1 tsp. low-fat mayonnaise
- 1 tbs. characteristic yogurt
- 1 tbs. rice vinegar
- 2 leaves mint, finely hacked
- Salt and newly ground dark pepper

Instruction

1 Preheat the grill to 200°C (180°C fan/Gas 6).

2 Place the salmon filet on a heating plate and prepare for 16–18 minutes until simply cooked through. Expel from the stove and put it in a safe spot. The salmon is similarly decent hot or cold in the plate of mixed greens. If your salmon has skin, basically cook skin side and expel the salmon from the skin utilizing a fish cut after cooking. It should slide off effectively when cooked.

3 In a little bowl, combine the mayonnaise, yogurt, rice wine vinegar, mint leaves, and salt and pepper and leave to represent at any rate 5 minutes to permit the flavors to create.

4 Arrange the plate of mixed greens leaves and spinach on a serving plate and top with the radishes, cucumber, spring onions, and parsley. Drop the cooked salmon onto the serving of mixed greens and shower the dressing over.

Choc Chip Granola

Chocolate at breakfast! Make certain to present with some green tea to give you a lot of SIRTs. The rice malt syrup can be subbed with maple syrup if you like.

Ingredients

- 200g enormous oats

- 50g walnuts, generally

- chopped

- 3 tbs. light olive oil

- 20g margarine

- 1 tbs. dim earthy colored sugar

- 2 tbs. rice malt syrup

- 60g great quality (70%)

- Dark chocolate chips

Instructions:

1 Preheat the grill to 160°C (140°C fan/Gas 3). Line a huge preparing plate with a silicone sheet or heating material.

2 Mix the oats and walnuts in an enormous bowl. In a little non-stick dish, tenderly heat the olive oil, spread, earthy colored sugar, and rice malt syrup until the margarine has

liquefied and the sugar and syrup have broken down. Try not to permit to bubble. Pour the syrup over the oats and mix completely until the oats are completely secured.

3 Distribute the granola over the heating plate, spreading directly into the corners. Leave clusters of blend with dividing instead of an even spread. Heat in the stove for 20 minutes until just tinged brilliant earthy colored at the edges. Expel from the broiler and leave to cool on the plate.

4 When cool, separate any greater bumps on the plate with your fingers and afterward blend in the chocolate chips. Scoop or empty the granola into a water/air proof tub or container.

Fragrant Asian Hotpot

Ingredients

- 1 tsp. tomato purée
- 1-star anise, squashed (or 1/4 tsp ground anise)

- Small bunch (10g) parsley, follows finely hacked

- Small bunch (1Og) coriander, follows finely hacked

- Juice of 1/2 lime

- 500ml chicken stock, new or made with one solid shape

- 1/2 carrot, stripped and cut into matchsticks

- 50g broccoli, cut into little florets

- 50g beansprouts

- 100g crude tiger prawns

- 100g firm tofu, hacked

- 50g rice noodles, cooked by parcel instructions

- 50g cooked water chestnuts, depleted

- 20g sushi ginger, hacked

- 1 tbs. great quality miso glue

Instructions:

Spot the tomato purée, star anise, parsley stalks, coriander stalks, lime juice, and chicken stock in a huge skillet and bring to a stew for 10 minutes.

Include the carrot, broccoli, prawns, tofu, noodles, and water chestnuts and stew delicately until the prawns are cooked through. Expel from the heat and mix in the sushi ginger and miso glue.

Serve with the coriander leaves and parsley.

Butternut Squash and Date Tagine

Staggering warming Moroccan flavors make this healthy tagine ideal for cold harvest time and winter nighttimes. Present with buckwheat for an additional wellbeing kick!

Ingredients

- 2 tablespoons olive oil
- 1 red onion, cut
- 2cm ginger, ground
- 3 garlic cloves, ground or squashed
- 1 teaspoon bean stew pieces (or to taste)
- 2 teaspoons cumin seeds
- 1 cinnamon stick
- 2 teaspoons ground turmeric

- 800g sheep neck filet, cut into 2cm pieces

- ½ teaspoon salt

- 100g Medjool dates, hollowed and cleaved

- 400g tin cleaved tomatoes, in addition to a large portion of a container of water

- 500g butternut squash, cleaved into 1cm 3D shapes

- 400g tin chickpeas, depleted

- 2 tablespoons new coriander (in addition to extra for embellishing)

- Buckwheat, couscous, flatbreads or rice to serve

Instructions:

1. Preheat your stove to 140C.

2. Shower around two tablespoons of olive oil into a huge ovenproof pan or cast iron meal dish. Include the cut onion and cook on a delicate heat, with the cover on, for around 5 minutes, until the onions are mollified yet not earthy colored.

3. Include the ground garlic and ginger, bean stew, cumin, cinnamon, and turmeric. Mix well and cook for one progressively minute with the top off. Include a sprinkle of

water if it gets excessively dry.

4. Next include the sheep lumps. Mix well to cover the meat in the onions and flavors and afterward include the salt, hacked dates, and tomatoes, in addition to about a large portion of a jar of water (100-200ml).

5. Bring the tagine to the bubble and afterward put the top on and put in your preheated grill for 1 hour and 15 minutes.

6. Thirty minutes before the finish of the cooking time, include the cleaved butternut squash and depleted chickpeas. Mix everything, set the top back on, and come back to the stove for the last 30 minutes of cooking.

7. When the tagine is prepared, expel from the stove and mix through the slashed coriander. Present with buckwheat, couscous, flatbreads, or basmati rice.

If you don't claim an ovenproof pan or cast iron goulash dish, essentially cook the tagine in an ordinary pot up until it needs to go in the stove and afterward move the tagine into a customary lidded meal dish before setting in the appliance. Extra an additional 5 minutes of cooking time to take into consideration the way that the goulash dish will require additional opportunity to heat up.

Prawn Arrabbiata

Ingredients

- 125-150 g Raw or cooked prawns (Ideally lord prawns)

- 65 g Buckwheat pasta

- 1 tbs. extra virgin olive oil

For the arrabbiata sauce

- 40 g Red onion, finely hacked

- 1 Garlic clove, finely hacked

- 30 g Celery, finely hacked

- 1 Bird's eye stew, finely hacked

- 1 tsp. Dried blended herbs

- 1 tsp. extra virgin olive oil

- 2 tbs. White wine (discretionary)

- 400 g Tinned hacked tomatoes

- 1 tbs. Chopped parsley

Instructions:

1. Fry the onion, garlic, celery, and stew and dried herbs in the oil over medium-low heat for 1–2 minutes. Turn the heat up

to medium, include the wine, and cook for one moment. Include the tomatoes and leave the sauce to stew over medium-low heat for 20–30 minutes, until it has a pleasant rich consistency.

2. While the sauce is cooking, carry a skillet of water to the bubble and cook the pasta as indicated by the bundle instructions. At the point when cooked just as you would prefer, channel, hurl with the olive oil and keep in the container until required.

3. If you are utilizing crude prawns, add them to the sauce and cook for a further 3–4 minutes until they have turned pink and dark, include the parsley and serve. If you are utilizing cooked prawns, include them with the parsley, carry the sauce to the bubble and serve.

4. Add the cooked pasta to the sauce, blend completely yet tenderly and serve.

Turmeric Baked Salmon

Ingredients

- 125-150 g Skinned Salmon

- 1 tsp. extra virgin olive oil

- 1 tsp. Ground turmeric

- 1/4 Juice of a lemon

For the zesty celery

- 1 tsp. extra virgin olive oil

- 40 g Red onion, finely cleaved

- 60 g Tinned green lentils

- 1 Garlic clove, finely cleaved

- 1 cm Fresh ginger, finely cleaved

- 1 Bire's eye stew, finely slashed

- 150 g Celery, cut into 2cm lengths

- 1 tsp Mild curry powder

- 130 g Tomato, cut into eight wedges

- 100 ml Chicken or vegetable stock

- 1 tbsp. Chopped parsley

Instructions:

Heat the stove to 200C/gas mark 6.

Start with the hot celery. Heat a skillet over medium-low heat, including the olive oil, at that point the onion, garlic, ginger, bean stew, and celery. Fry delicately for 2–3 minutes or until mellowed; however not hued, at that point, include the curry powder and cook for a further moment.

Include the tomatoes, then the stock and lentils, and stew tenderly for 10 minutes. You might need to increment or reduction the cooking time contingent upon how crunchy you like your celery.

Then, blend the turmeric, oil, and lemon squeeze and rub over the salmon— Place on a heating plate and cook for 8–10 minutes.

To complete, mix the parsley through the celery and present it with the salmon.

Crowning Ceremony Chicken Salad

Ingredients

- 75 g Natural yogurt

- Juice of 1/4 of a lemon

- 1 tsp. Coriander

- 1 tsp. Ground turmeric

- 1/2 tsp. Mild curry powder

- 100 g Cooked chicken bosom, cut into reduced pieces

- 6 Walnut parts, finely slashed

- 1 Medjool date, finely slashed

- 20 g Red onion, diced

- 1 Bird's eye bean stew

- 40 g Rocket, to serve

Instructions:

Blend the yogurt, lemon juice, coriander, and flavors in a bowl. Include all the rest of the ingredients and serve on a bed of the rocket.

Heated Potatoes with Spicy Chickpea Stew-Sirtfood Recipes

Sort of Mexican Mole meets North African Tagine, this Spicy Chickpea Stew is inconceivably delectable and makes a great garnish for heated potatoes, in addition to it simply happens to be veggie lover, vegetarian, gluten-free and dairy-free. What's more, it contains chocolate.

Ingredients

- 4-6 heating potatoes, pricked everywhere

- 2 tablespoons olive oil

- 2 red onions, finely slashed

- 4 cloves garlic, ground or squashed

- 2cm ginger, ground

- ½ - 2 teaspoons bean stew pieces (contingent upon how hot you like things)

- 2 tablespoons cumin seeds

- 2 tablespoons turmeric

- Splash of water

- 2 x 400g tins cleaved tomatoes.

- 2 x 400g tins of chickpeas, including the chickpea water.

- 2 yellow peppers (or whatever shading you like!), cleaved into bitesize pieces

- 2 tablespoons parsley in addition to extra for embellish

- Salt and pepper to taste (discretionary)

- Side plate of mixed greens (discretionary)

Instructions:

1. Preheat the stove to 200C; in the meantime, you can set up the entirety of your ingredients.

2. At the point when the appliance is hot enough, place your heating potatoes in the stove and cook for 1 hour or until they are done how you like them.

3. When the potatoes are in the stove, place the olive oil and slashed red onion in a huge wide pot and cook tenderly, with the cover on for 5 minutes, until the onions are delicate however not earthy colored.

4. Evacuate the cover and include the garlic, ginger, cumin, and bean stew. Cook for a further moment on low heat; at that point, include the turmeric and an exceptionally little sprinkle of water and cook for one more moment, taking consideration not to let the skillet get excessively dry.

5. Next, include the tomatoes, cocoa powder (or cacao), chickpeas (counting the chickpea water), and yellow pepper. Stew on a low heat for 45 minutes until the sauce is thick and greasy (yet don't allow it to consume!). The stew ought to be done at generally a similar time as the potatoes.

6. At long last mix in the two tablespoons of parsley, and some salt and pepper if you wish, and serve the stew on the heated potatoes, maybe with a basic side plate of mixed greens.

Red Onion Dhal and Kale with Buckwheat-Sirtfood

Flavorful and extremely nutritious, this Kale and Red Onion

Dhal with Buckwheat is fast and simple to make and normally gluten-free, dairy-free, veggie lover, and vegetarian.

Ingredients

- 1 tablespoon olive oil

- 1 little red onion, cut

- 3 garlic cloves, ground or squashed

- 2 cm ginger, ground

- 1 feathered creatures' eye stew, deseeded and finely cleaved

- 2 teaspoons of turmeric

- 2 teaspoons of masala

- 150g red lentils

- 500ml of coconut milk

- 200ml water

- 100g of kale

- 160g buckwheat (or earthy colored rice)

Instructions:

1. Put the olive oil in an enormous, profound pan and include the cut onion. Cook on low heat, with the cover on for 5 minutes until mollified.

2. Include the garlic, ginger, and bean stew and cook for brief more.

3. Include the turmeric, garam masala, and a sprinkle of water and cook for one increasingly minute.

4. Include the red lentils, coconut milk, and 200ml water (do this essentially considerably filling the coconut milk can with water and tipping it into the pan).

5. Combine everything all together and cook for 20 minutes over a tenderly heat with the cover on. Mix periodically and include somewhat more water if the dhal begins to stick.

6. Following 20 minutes include the kale, mix all together and supplant the cover, cook for a further 5 minutes (1-2 minutes if you use spinach!)

7. Around 15 minutes before the curry is prepared, place the buckwheat in a medium pot and include a lot of bubbling

water. Take the water back to the bubble and cook for 10 minutes (or somewhat more if you incline toward your buckwheat milder.

Chargrilled Beef with Garlic Kale, a Red Wine Jus, Onion Rings, and Herb Roasted Potatoes-Sirtfood

Ingredients:

- 80g potatoes, stripped and cut into 2cm bones

- 1 tsp. additional virgin olive oil

- 5g parsley, finely slashed

- 50g red onion, cut into rings

- 50g kale, cut

- 1 garlic clove, finely slashed

- 120–150g x 3.5cm-thick hamburger filet steak or 2cm-thick sirloin steak

- 40ml red wine

- 150ml hamburger stock

- 1 tsp. tomato purée

- 1 tsp. Cornflour disintegrated in 1 tsp. water

Instructions:

- Heat the grill to 220ºC/gas 7.

- Place the potatoes in a pan of bubbling water, take back to the bubble and cook for 4–5 minutes, at that point channel. Spot in a cooking tin with one teaspoon of the oil and meal in the hot stove for 35–45 minutes. Turn the potatoes at regular intervals to guarantee in any event, cooking. At the point when cooked, expel from the broiler, sprinkle with the slashed parsley, and blend.

- Now, fry the onion in the oil over a normal heat for about 7 minutes, until delicate and pleasantly caramelized. Keep warm. Steam the kale for 2–3 minutes at that point channel. Fry the garlic tenderly in ½ teaspoon of oil for one moment, until delicate however not shaded. Include the kale and fry for a further 1–2 minutes, until delicate. Keep warm.

- Heat an ovenproof skillet over high heat until smoking. Have the meat placed in a teaspoon of the oil and fry in the hot skillet over medium-high heat, as indicated by how you like your meat done. If you like your meat medium, it is smarter to burn the meat and afterward move the container to a stove set at 220ºC/gas seven and finish the cooking that path for the recommended occasions.

- Remove the meat from the dish and put aside to rest. Add wine to the hot skillet to raise any meat buildup. Air pocket to diminish the wine considerably.

- Add the tomato purée to the steak dish and bring to the bubble; at that point, add the cornflour glue to thicken your sauce, including it a little at once until you have your ideal consistency. Mix in any of the juices from the refreshed steak and present with the broiled potatoes, kale, onion rings, and red wine sauce.

Kale and Blackcurrant Smoothie

Ingredients

- 2 tsp nectar
- 1 cup newly made green tea

- 10 child kale leaves, stalks expelled

- 1 ready banana

- 40 g blackcurrants

- 6 ice 3D shapes

Instruction

Mix the nectar into the warm green tea until it breaks. Marvel all the ingredients together in a blender until smooth. Serve right away.

Buckwheat Pasta Salad

Ingredients

- 50g buckwheat pasta (cooked by the bundle instructions)

- Large bunch of rocket

- Small bunch of basil leaves

- 8 cherry tomatoes, split

- 1/2 avocado, diced

- 10 olives

- 1 tbs. additional virgin olive oil

- 20g pine nuts

Delicately join all the ingredients aside from the pine nuts and mastermind on a plate or in a bowl; at that point, disperse the pine nuts over the top.

Greek Salad Skewers

Ingredients

- 2 wooden sticks, absorbed water for 30 minutes before use

- 8 enormous dark olives

- 8 cherry tomatoes

- 1 yellow pepper, cut into eight squares

- ½ red onion cut the middle and isolated into eight pieces

- 100g (about 10cm) cucumber, cut into four cuts and split

- 100g feta, cut into eight 3D shapes

For the dressing:

- 1 tbs. additional virgin olive oil

- Juice of ½ lemon

- 1 tsp. balsamic vinegar

- ½ clove garlic, stripped and squashed

- Few leaves basil, finely cleaved (or ½ tsp dried blended herbs to supplant basil and oregano)

- Few leaves oregano, finely cleaved

Liberal flavoring of salt and newly ground dark pepper

Instruction

1 Thread each stick with the serving of mixed greens ingredients in the request: olive, tomato, yellow pepper, red onion, cucumber, feta, tomato, olive, yellow pepper, red onion, cucumber, feta.

2 Place all the dressing ingredients in a little bowl and combine it all. Pour over the sticks.

Kale, Edamame and Tofu Curry

Ingredients

- 1 tbs. rapeseed oil

- 1 huge onion, slashed

- 4 cloves garlic, stripped and ground

- 1 huge thumb (7cm) new ginger, stripped and ground

- 1 red stew, deseeded and meagerly cut

- 1/2 tsp. ground turmeric

- 1/4 tsp. cayenne pepper

- 1 tsp. paprika

- 1/2 tsp. ground cumin

- 1 tsp. salt

- 250g dried red lentils

- 1-liter bubbling water

- 50g solidified soyaedamame beans

- 200g firm tofu, hacked into shapes

- 2 tomatoes, generally hacked

- Juice of 1 lime

- 200g kale leaves stalks evacuated and torn

Instructions:

1 Put the oil in an overwhelming bottomed container over

low-medium heat. Include the onion and cook for 5 minutes before including the garlic, ginger, and stew and cooking for a further 2 minutes. Include turmeric, cayenne, paprika, cumin, and salt. Mix through before including the red lentils and blending once more.

2 Pour in the bubbling water and bring to a healthy stew for 10 minutes; at that point, diminish the heat and cook for about 30 minutes until the curry has a thick porridge feel.

3 Add the tofu, soya beans, and tomatoes and cook for an extra 5 minutes. Include the lime juice and kale leaves and cook until the kale is simply delicate.

Chocolate Cupcakes with Matcha Icing

Ingredients
- 150g self-rising flour
- 200g caster sugar
- 60g cocoa
- ½ tsp. salt

- ½ tsp. fine coffee espresso, decaf whenever liked

- 120ml milk

- ½ tsp. vanilla concentrate

- 50ml vegetable oil

- 1 egg

- 120ml bubbling water

- For the icing:

- 50g spread, at room temperature

- 50g icing sugar

- 1 tsp. matcha green tea powder

- ½ tsp. vanilla bean glue

- 50g delicate cream cheddar

Instruction

• Place a cupcake tin with paper or silicone cake cases.

• Place the cocoa, flour, salt, sugar, and coffee powder in a huge bowl and blend completely.

• Add the milk, vanilla concentrate, vegetable oil, and egg to the dry ingredients and utilize an electric blender to beat until all-around joined. Cautiously pour in the bubbling water gradually and beat on low speed until completely consolidated. Utilize a rapid to beat for a further moment to add air to the player. The hitter is significantly more fluid than a typical cake blend. Have confidence, and it will taste astonishing!

• Spoon the hitter equitably between the cake cases. Each cake case ought to be close to ¾ full. Prepare in the grill for 15-18 minutes, until the blend bobs back when tapped. Expel from the stove and permit to cool totally before icing.

• To make the icing, cream the spread and icing sugar together until it's pale and smooth. Include the matcha powder and vanilla and mix once more. At last, include the cream cheddar and beat until smooth. Channel or spread over the cakes.

Sesame Chicken Salad

Ingredients

•   1 tbs. sesame seeds

•   1 cucumber, stripped, divided lengthways, deseeded with a teaspoon and cut

•   100g child kale, generally cleaved

- 60g pak choi, finely destroyed

- ½ red onion, finely cut

- Large bunch (20g) parsley, cleaved

- 150g cooked chicken, destroyed

For the dressing:

- 1 tsp. additional virgin olive oil

- 1 tsp. sesame oil

- Juice of 1 lime

- 1 tsp. clear nectar

- 2 tsp. soy sauce

Instruction

1. Fry the sesame in a dry skillet for about 2 minutes until daintily seared and fragrant. Move to a plate to cool.

2. In a little bowl, combine the olive oil, sesame oil, lime juice, nectar, and soy sauce.

3 Place the pak choi, red onion, cucumber, kale, and parsley in a huge bowl and tenderly combine. Pour over the dressing

and blend once more.

4 Distribute the serving of mixed greens between two plates and top with the destroyed chicken. Sprinkle over the sesame seeds not long before serving.

Sirtfood Mushroom Scramble Eggs

Ingredients

- 2 eggs
- 1 tsp. ground turmeric
- 1 tsp. gentle curry powder
- 20g kale, generally cleaved
- 1 tsp. additional virgin olive oil
- Handful of catch mushrooms, daintily cut
- 5g parsley, finely hacked
- Add a seed blend as a topper and some Rooster Sauce for flavor (optional)

Instructions

Blend the turmeric and curry powder and include a little

water until you have accomplished a light glue.

Steam the kale for 2–3 minutes.

Heat the oil in a skillet over medium heat and fry the bean stew and mushrooms for 2–3 minutes until they have begun to brand relax.

Sweet-smelling Chicken Breast with Kale, Red Onion, and Salsa

Ingredients:

- 120g skinless, boneless chicken bosom
- 2 tsp ground turmeric
- Juice of ¼ lemon
- 1 tsp. additional virgin olive oil
- 50g kale, slashed
- 20g red onion, cut
- 1 tsp. slashed new ginger
- 50g buckwheat

Instructions:

To make the salsa, expel the eye from the tomato and slash it finely, taking consideration to keep however much of the fluid as could be expected. Blend in with the stew, tricks, parsley, and lemon juice. You could place everything in a blender, yet the final product is somewhat unique.

Heat the grill to 220ºC/gas 7. Marinate the chicken bosom in 1 teaspoon of the turmeric, the lemon juice, and a little oil. Leave for 5–10 minutes.

Heat an ovenproof skillet until hot, at that point include the marinated chicken and cook for a moment or so on each side, until pale brilliant, at that point move to the stove (place on a preparing plate if your container isn't ovenproof) for 8–10 minutes or until cooked through. Expel from the stove, spread with foil and leave to rest for 5 minutes before serving.

Then, cook the kale in a liner for about 5 minutes. Then, fry the red onions and the ginger in a little oil, until delicate yet not shaded, at that point include the cooked kale and fry for one more moment.

Cook the buckwheat as indicated by the parcel instructions with the rest of the teaspoon of turmeric. Serve nearby the chicken, vegetables, and salsa.

Smoked Salmon Omelet

Attempt this fast and simple Sirtfood dish pressed with flavor and goodness.

Ingredients

- 2 Medium eggs
- 100 g Smoked salmon, cut
- 1/2 tsp. Capers
- 10 g Rocket, cleaved
- 1 tsp. Parsley, cleaved
- 1 tsp. extra virgin olive oil

Instructions:

Whisk the eggs into a bowl very well after breaking them. Include the salmon, escapades, rocket, and parsley.

Heat the olive oil in a non-stick skillet until hot, however not smoking. Include the egg blend and, utilizing a spatula or fish cut, move the blend around the container until it is even. Diminish the heat and let the omelet cook through. Slide the spatula around the edges and move up or overlap the omelet in the middle of serving.

Green Tea Smoothie

This super-healthy smoothie utilizes matcha powder, which is an exceptionally thought Japanese green tea. It very well may be found in authority Asian or coffee bars.

Ingredients

- 2 ready bananas
- 250 ml milk
- 2 tsp. matcha green tea powder
- 1/2 tsp. vanilla bean glue (not extricate) or a little

scratch of the seeds from a vanilla unit

- 6 ice 3D shapes

- 2 tsp. nectar

Instruction

Mix every of the ingredients in a blender and serve as desired.

Sirtfood Marinated Cod with Sesame

Ingredients

- 20g miso

- 1 tbsp mirin

- 1 tbsp additional virgin olive oil

- 200g skinless cod filet

- 20g red onion, cut

- 40g celery, cut

- 1 garlic clove, finely hacked

- 1 10,000 foot stew, finely slashed

- 1 tsp finely hacked new ginger

- 60g green beans

- 50g kale, generally hacked

- 1 tsp sesame seeds

- 5g parsley, generally hacked

- 1 tbsp tamari

- 30g buckwheat

- 1 tsp ground turmeric

Instructions

Blend the miso, mirin, and one teaspoon of the oil. Rub everywhere throughout the cod and leave to marinate for 30 minutes. Heat the stove to 220ºC/gas 7.

Prepare the cod for 10 minutes.

In the interim, heat a huge skillet or wok with the rest of the oil. Include the onion and pan-fried food for a couple of moments; at that point, include the celery, garlic, stew, ginger, green beans, and kale. Hurl and fry until the kale is delicate and cooked through.

Cook the buckwheat as per the bundle instructions with the turmeric for 3 minutes.

Include the sesame seeds, parsley, and tamari to the pan-fried food and present with the greens and fish.

Raspberry and Blackcurrant Jelly

Making a jam ahead of time is a great method to set up the natural product with the goal that it is prepared to eat before anything else.

Ingredients

- 100g raspberries washed
- 2 leaves gelatine
- 100g blackcurrants washed and follows expelled
- 2 tbsp granulated sugar
- 300ml water

Instruction

1 Place the raspberries in two separate serving dishes/glasses/molds.

2 Place the blackcurrants in a little dish with the sugar and 100ml water and bring it to the bubble. Stew energetically for

5 minutes and afterward expel from the heat. Leave to represent 2 minutes.

3 Squeeze out overabundance water from the gelatine leaves and add them to the pot. Mix until completely broken down, at that point mix in the remainder of the water. Empty the fluid into the readied dishes and refrigerate to set. The jams ought to be prepared in around 3-4 hours or overnight.

Apple Pancakes with Blackcurrant Compote

Ingredients

- 75g porridge oats

- 125g plain flour

- 1 tsp. heating powder

- 2 tsp. caster sugar

- Pinch of salt

- 2 apples, stripped, cored and cut into little pieces

- 300ml semi-skimmed milk

- 2 egg whites

- 2 tsp. light olive oil

For the compote:

- 120g blackcurrants washed and followed evacuated
- 2 tsp. caster sugar
- 3 tsp. water

Instruction

1 First, make the compote. Spot the blackcurrants, sugar, and water in a little skillet. Raise to a stew and cook for 10-15 minutes.

2 Place the oats, flour, heating powder, caster sugar and salt in a huge bowl and blend well. Mix in the apple and afterward race in the milk a little at once until you have a smooth blend. Whisk the egg whites to hardened pinnacles and afterward overlay into the flapjack hitter. Move the player to a container.

3 Heat the oil in a non-stick skillet on medium-high heat and pour in roughly one-fourth of the player. Cook on the two sides until brilliant earthy colored. Expel and repeat to make four hotcakes.

4 Serve the hotcakes with the blackcurrant compote sprinkled over.

Sirt Fruit Salad

Ingredients

- ½ cup newly made green tea

- 1 tsp. nectar

- 1 orange, split

- 1 apple, cored and generally cleaved

- 10 red seedless grapes

- 10 blueberries

Instructions:

1. Mix the nectar into a large portion of some green tea, at the point when broken down, including the juice of a large portion of the orange. Leave to cool.

2. Hack the other portion of the orange and spot in a bowl along with the slashed apple, grapes, and blueberries. Pour

over the cooled tea and leave to soak for a couple of moments before serving.

Sirtfood Bites

Ingredients

- 120g pecans

- 30g dull chocolate (85 percent cocoa solids), broken into pieces; or cocoa nibs

- 250g Medjool dates pitted

- 1 tsp. cocoa powder

- 1 tsp. ground turmeric

- 1 tsp. additional virgin olive oil

- The scratched seeds of one vanilla case or 1 tsp vanilla concentrate

- 1–2 tsp. water

Instructions

- Place the pecans and chocolate in a food processor and procedure until you have a fine powder.

- Add the various ingredients aside from the water and mix until the blend shapes a ball. You could conceivably need to include the water depending on the consistency of the blend – you don't need it to be excessively clingy.

- Using your hands, structure the blend into reduced balls and refrigerate in a hermetically sealed compartment for at any rate one hour before eating them.

- You could move a portion of the balls in some more cocoa or dried up a coconut to accomplish an alternate completion if you like.

- They will keep for as long as one week in your refrigerator.

Sirt Muesli

Ingredients:

- 20g buckwheat chips
- 10g buckwheat puffs

- 15g coconut chips or dried up coconut

- 40g Medjool dates, hollowed and hacked

- 15g pecans, hacked

- 10g cocoa nibs

- 100g strawberries, hulled and hacked

- 100g plain Greek yogurt (or veggie lover elective, for example, soya or coconut yogurt)

Instructions:

Blend the entirety of the above ingredients, possibly including the yogurt and strawberries before serving if you are making it in mass.

Chinese-Style Pork with Pak Choi

Ingredients

- 400g firm tofu, cut into enormous 3D squares

- 1 tsp. cornflour sirtfood recipes

- 1 tsp. water

- 125ml chicken stock

- 1 tsp. rice wine

- 1 tsp. tomato purée

- 1 tsp. earthy colored sugar

- 1 tsp. soy sauce

- 1 clove garlic, stripped and squashed

- 1 thumb (5cm) new ginger, stripped and ground 1 tbsp rapeseed oil

- 100g shiitake mushrooms, cut

- 1 shallot, stripped and cut

- 200g pak choi or choi aggregate, cut into dainty cuts 400g pork mince (10% fat)

- 100g beansprouts

- Large bunch (20g) parsley, cleaved

Here's the secret:

- Lay out the tofu on kitchen paper, spread with more kitchen paper, and put in a safe spot.

- In a little bowl, combine the cornflour and water, evacuating all protuberances. Include the chicken stock, rice wine, tomato purée, earthy colored sugar, and soy sauce. Include the squashed garlic and ginger and mix.

•	In a wok or enormous skillet, heat the oil to a high temperature. Include the shiitake mushrooms and pan-fried food for 2–3 minutes until cooked and glossy. Expel the mushrooms from the dish with an opened spoon and put it in a safe spot. Add the tofu to the dish and pan-fried food until brilliant on all sides. Expel with an opened spoon and put it in a safe spot.

•	Add the shallot and pak choi to the wok, pan sear for 2 minutes, at that point, include the mince. Cook until the mince is cooked through; at that point, include the sauce, lessen the heat an indent, and permit the sauce to rise round the meat for a moment or two. Include the beansprouts, shiitake mushrooms, and tofu to the skillet and warm through. Expel from the heat, mix through the parsley, and serve right away.

Tuscan Bean Stew

Instructions:

•	1 tsp. additional virgin olive oil

- 50g red onion, finely slashed

- 30g carrot, stripped and finely chopped sirtfood recipes

- 30g celery, cut and finely slashed

- 1 garlic clove, finely slashed

- ½ superior bean stew, finely slashed (discretionary)

- 1 tsp. herbes de Provence

- 200ml vegetable stock

- 1 x 400g tin slashed Italian tomatoes

- 1 tsp. tomato purée

- 200g tinned blended beans

- 50g kale, generally slashed

- 1 tsp. generally slashed parsley

- 40g buckwheat

Method

Spot the oil in a medium pan over low–medium heat and delicately fry the onion, carrot, celery, garlic, chili (if utilizing) and herbs, until the onion is delicate, however not shaded.

Include the stock, tomatoes and tomato purée and bring to the bubble. Include the beans and stew for 30 minutes.

Include the kale and cook for another 5–10 minutes until delicate, at that point, include the parsley.

In the meantime, cook the buckwheat as indicated by the bundle instructions, channel, and afterward present with the stew.

The Sirtfood diet rest on the fact that specific foods initiate sirtuins in your bo
which are specific proteins theorized to receive different rewards, from shieldi
cells in your body from inflammation to turning around maturing. Foods permitt
on a diet incorporate green tea, dim chocolate, apples, natural citrus produc
parsley, turmeric, kale, blueberries, tricks, and red wine. At the point when y
follow the Sirtfood diet, you'll start with phase 1—which goes on for seven da
During the initial three days of the menu, you'll drink three Sirtfood juices and ha
one Sirtfood-rich meal for a day by day aggregate of 1,000 calori
On days four through the seventh day, you'll expend 1,500 complete calories, dri
two green squeezes and eat two healthy Sirtfood-rich meals. This finishes at pha
1. Phase 2 keeps going 14 days and permits you to eat three adjusted Sirtfood-ri
meals and one green juice day by day. After phase 2 is finished, you'll follow an i
creasingly typical method of eating—yet are urged to fuse sirtuin-initiating foo
into ordinary meal plans. You can retake phases 1 and 2 whenever you have to lo
more   weight   or   muscle   to   fat   rat

TOXIC AMERICA

ESSAYS

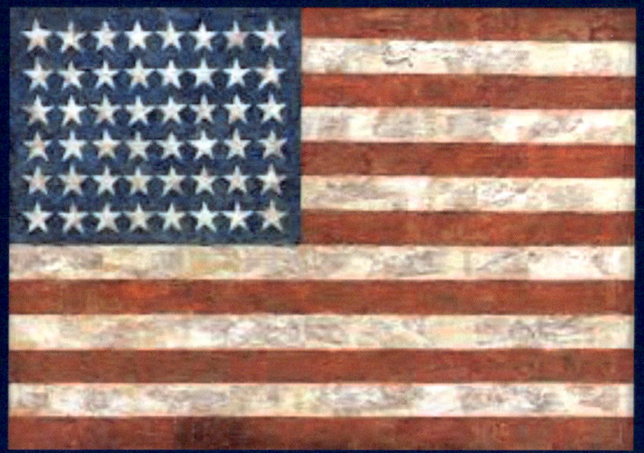

J.D. GILL PH.D